Métis Coming Together

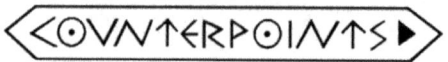

Shirley R. Steinberg
Series Editor

Vol. 557

Métis Coming Together

SHARING OUR STORIES AND KNOWLEDGES

Edited by
Laura Forsythe and Jennifer Markides

PETER LANG
New York · Berlin · Bruxelles · Chennai · Lausanne · Oxford

Library of Congress Cataloging-in-Publication Control Number: 2024946937

Bibliographic information published by the Deutsche Nationalbibliothek.
The German National Library lists this publication in the German
National Bibliography; detailed bibliographic data is available
on the Internet at http://dnb.d-nb.de.

Cover design by Peter Lang Group AG

ISSN 1058-1634 (print)
ISBN 9783034354042 (paperback)
ISBN 9783034353205 (hardback)
ISBN 9783034354028 (ebook)
ISBN 9783034354035 (epub)
DOI 10.3726/b22355

© 2025 Peter Lang Group AG, Lausanne
Published by Peter Lang Publishing Inc., New York, USA
info@peterlang.com— www.peterlang.com

All rights reserved.
All parts of this publication are protected by copyright.
Any utilization outside the strict limits of the copyright law, without the permission of the publisher, is forbidden and liable to prosecution.
This applies in particular to reproductions, translations, microfilming, and storage and processing in electronic retrieval systems.

This publication has been peer reviewed.

TABLE OF CONTENTS

Foreword   ix
Chelsea Gabel

Introduction: Multifaceted Métis: Unavoidable
Considerations Around Our Complex Identities   1
Jennifer Markides and Laura Forsythe

1   The Reason We Gather: Métis-Specific Spaces   7
Laura Forsythe and Lucy Delgado

2   Red River Readers in Multivocal Flux: Across, Between,
and Beyond Traditional Disciplinary Approaches to Métis
Studies   19
Red River Readers

3   The Power of Dancing in Two Worlds: Finding a Fit for
Métis Identities in Academia   35
Shannon Leddy

	TABLE OF CONTENTS	
4	The Métis Nation, Epistemic Injustice, and Self-Indigenization *Kurtis Boyer and Paul Simard Smith*	45
5	Returning to Ceremony: A Métis Spiritual Resurgence *Chantal Fiola*	57
6	Archaeology with Our Ancestors: The Exploring Métis Identity Through Archaeology (EMITA) Project *Kisha Supernant, Emily Haines, Solène Mallet Gauthier, Maria Nelson, Eric Tebby, William T. D. Wadsworth and Dawn Wambold*	71
7	On Being Elsewhere to Stay: Reflections on Métis Responsibilities Living in the Homelands of Other People *Robert L. A. Hancock*	89
8	"It's Very Different Walking in Two Worlds as a Métis Person": Identity, Community, Culture and Connections as Determinants of the Health and Wellbeing of Métis Peoples *Heather Foulds, Jamie LaFleur and Leah Ferguson*	97
9	The Grandmothers of the Prairies to Woodlands Indigenous Language Revitalization Circle *Laura Forsythe*	117
10	*Li Keur, Riel's Heart of the North*, an Artistic Narration of Métis History through Peoplehood: Addressing Métis (mis)Recognition and Recentering Métis Women *Suzanne M. Steele, with an introduction by Nicole Stonyk*	131
11	Métis Arts as Education: Visual Storytelling, and More, in Alberta *Yvonne Poitras Pratt and Billie-Jo Grant*	149

12	Raindrops, Fiddles, and Tall Tales: Navigating Our Diversity Through Storytelling *Angie Tucker*	161
13	Learning to Listen Closely: The Listening Guide and "I Poems" in Métis Research Methodologies *Lucy Delgado*	169
14	I Could Turn into a River When I Was a Girl: Crooked Methodologies and the Gathering Research Framework *Michelle Porter*	177
15	Storying Métis Sexualities: Métis Confessions: Our First Time—Red River Edition *Angie Tucker, KD King (Sangria Jiggz), Tanya Ball and Paul L. Gareau*	187

FOREWORD
Chelsea Gabel

Who are the Métis? Are you really Métis? How Indigenous are you really? These are questions often directed at and about Métis people. Such questions continue to be asked as ways to affirm or challenge our experience of being or our right to exist in relation to First Nations and Inuit peoples. At the same time, we have seen a ripple effect of non-Métis claiming to be Métis while asserting our identities to increase their own connections to the land and resources. Coupled together, these thoughts and actions have helped obfuscate Métis identity and experiences of being.

I would be remiss in writing a foreword for a book on Métis identity without declaring my own. I am Métis from Rivers, Manitoba, and spent much of my childhood and youth in Winnipeg—the heart of the Métis homeland—before moving to Ontario, where I currently reside and work as a professor in the Department of Health, Aging and Society and the Indigenous Studies Department at McMaster University in Hamilton. I am a Desjarlais, a Fleury, and a card-carrying citizen of the Manitoba Métis Federation (MMF). My role in identity debates and spaces is deeply personal, as I was part of the small group of mostly Métis academics who filed a complaint of research misconduct against Carrie Bourassa in 2021. The news of Bourassa's identity fraud caused tremendous sadness, hurt, and feelings of betrayal, especially within the Métis community. Little did we know that the complaint and the CBC news story that followed would change identity politics in this country forever. In her interview with Robert Henry on Indigenous identity fraud, Caroline Tait (2023) argues that "what we need is a stronger collective voice" (p. 92). Thus, the arrival of *Métis Coming Together* by Jennifer Markides and Laura Forsythe is particularly timely and even more critical because it fulfills the mission in its title; it brings a strong collective Métis voice from those who have generously shared their knowledge and experiences about what it means to be Métis.

In Canada's body politic, Indigeneity is largely understood through a First Nations lens based on fragmented and often fictional understandings of the Indian Act (Kelm & Smith, 2018). Centering Indigeneity in the Indian Act erases Métis lived experiences and realities (Gaudry, 2018) including those of land dispossession (Teillet, 2019), the residential school system (TRC, 2015), the Sixties Scoop (Stevenson, 2019), and the half-breed scrip system (Graham & Davoren, 2015). Métis histories are most often framed around the Red River Resistance (1870) and the Northwest Resistance (1885). This perspective omits the distinct experiences of Métis histories such as Métis farms (Barron, 1990), Road Allowance communities (Barron, 1990; Quiring, 2003; Teillet, 2019), and Métis settlements (Mcdougall, 2017). The exclusion of Métis experiences from the broader Indigenous discourse has caused Métis to have to fight for recognition in any number of spaces, including academic spaces, that were created to include them under catch-all terminology such as "Aboriginal" and now "Indigenous." The effects of these experiences continue to implicate Métis not only intergenerationally but also politically. Our complex history and lack of recognition require understandings that extend beyond a one-size-fits-all approach to Indigenous relations and reconciliation, including recent efforts pointing to the need for distinctions-based approaches that honor the unique needs, experiences, and circumstances of the Métis (Nychuk, 2024).

The dominant narratives in Canada regarding the Métis center on historical and legal interpretations of Métis rather than an exploration of how Métis understand themselves in contemporary contexts. Colonization and settler colonialism have impacted how some of us have come to relate to our Métis identities, families, and communities. Some are forced to hide in plain sight as a form of protection, while others have continued to publicly fight for Métis rights. In all cases, Métis understandings of being have been and continue to be passed down intergenerationally, emphasizing our connections and distinctions as a people. Métis life is complex, yet at the same time it is simple.

Métis Coming Together looks to address that reality by providing insights into the various ways in which Métis people understand and express their identity today. This book further seeks to engage in research that is meaningful to Métis people and the communities they live in today.

In the powerful chapters that follow, readers will encounter a rich tapestry of stories, insights, and reflections that shed light on the diverse experiences of Métis people. We are neither the forgotten people that has so often been portrayed nor a mixture of First Nations and Europeans. *Métis Coming Together* honors the bravery, resilience, and strength of our people and is a testament to Métis people who have overcome adversity with grace, dignity, and unwavering determination. These are the stories of the Métis.

INTRODUCTION

Multifaceted Métis: Unavoidable Considerations Around Our Complex Identities

Jennifer Markides and Laura Forsythe

This was not supposed to be a book about identity. It never is. However, everything we write about Métis people—our histories, experiences, epistemologies, methodologies, and lives—speaks to who we are. Métis identity and Métis-ness imbue the work in this collection, *Métis Coming Together*.

We begin by positioning ourselves, the way many of the book's chapters do. Many Indigenous scholars have explained the importance of this practice, as it brings us into relationship with each other and situates us in relation to our families, communities, contexts, and places (Absolon, 2011; Absolon & Willett, 2005; Adese et al., 2017; Graveline, 2000; Kovach, 2009, 2017, 2021; LaRocque, 1975; McGregor et al., 2018; Moreton-Robinson, 2017; Smith, 2012). In many cases, we find cousins or distant relations. Those who are knowledgeable about the family names associated with different locations will know how your Métis family fits into the larger fabric of our shared history. Because our Métis identity is often misrepresented, misunderstood, and at times co-opted, knowing and stating our family connections becomes a validating and member-checking process for being Métis.

As co-editor of this collection, I, Jennifer Markides, am honored to be entrusted with the contributions in this book. I am a recognized member of the Métis Nation of Alberta. Despite having citizenship, for a long time I felt a sense of not belonging in our Métis circles. I would share my family names of McKay, Favel, Ballendine, Linklater, and McDermott and rarely hear a connection. Only in the last year was I at a Métis scholar gathering and had a family story shared by Anna Corrigal-Flaminio. I found kin. The sensation of that moment was equal parts excitement, validation, and relief. The scrutiny we face in academic positions is justified and rigorous, yet also terrifying. We do not want to be mistaken or proven not to be Métis. What other scholars live like this? It is a constant cloud that looms in every space. Hiring committees are navigating the identity politics, universities are implementing newly hatched policies, and ultimately Indigenous scholars and staff are taxed with policing who is and who is not Indigenous—faculty, staff, and students alike. It is complicated but necessary considering the climate of pretendianism and fraud. Ugh.

Laura Forsythe d-ishinikaashon. My name is Laura Forsythe. Ma famii kawyesh Roostertown d-oshciwak. My family was from Rooster Town a long time ago. Anosh ma famii Winnipeg wikiwak. Today, my family lives in Winnipeg. Ma Parentii (my ancestors) are the Huppe, Ward, Berard, Morin, Lavallee, and Cyr. Niya en Michif. I am Métis from the Red River Settlement, and I grew up in the heart of the Métis Homeland, like the generations of women before me. My maternal great-grandmother Nora Berard was born in Rooster Town on land known as lot 31, owned by my ancestor Jean Baptiste Berard, and my lineage includes Joseph Huppe, who fought in the Victory of Frog Plain. I am a citizen of the Manitoba Métis Federation. This is my positionality and community connection statement. It is who I claim to be and who claims me.

Beyond positioning, many aspects of identity come to the fore in this book. Some are explicit, and some are tacit. To be clear, there is no singular Métis identity. We are not simply Métis by virtue of being born of an Indigenous and settler union. Métis are a distinct people, as recognized by the 2016 *Daniels v. Canada* decision. Historically, we became a people with our own language (Michif, with many regionally influenced dialects), culture, tradition, commerce (Shore, 2018), ceremonial practices, stories, governance systems, and political movements. Some of these aspects of our identities—in past and present contexts—are discussed in the chapters that await the reader. These terms do not bind us in the present day. Identities are complex and not measured by blood quantum, place, language retention, or simply enacting cultural tropes. We are modern-day Métis and embody multifaceted manifestations of Métis-ness.

While none of the chapters sets out to define who we are as Métis people, many give examples of how we should not be defined or limited by preconceived or ill-considered ideas about what makes a Métis person. We are not defined by our ability or inability to speak our language, yet language is essential to many (see Forsythe, Chapter Nine). We are not limited to a narrow scope of religious expression and certainly not one defined by Métis leadership (see Fiola, Chapter Five). We can participate in ceremony or not and still be Métis.

For most of our history, being Métis was a precarious existence without recognition as a distinct and sovereign people. We lived differently yet often alongside our First Nations kin. Moreover, we were subjected to many of the same racist policies and oppressive experiences, leading many people to play into Indigenous stereotypes when needed, as noted by the Red River Métis Readers (Chapter Two) or to pass as having settler origins when necessary. Even now, Métis identity is fraught with imposter syndrome, as described by Leddy (Chapter Three). We are working to uncover and recover our stories and histories, literally in the case of the archeological mapping of Métis cabins using modern technologies and fine-grained analysis (see Supernant, Haines, Mallet Gauthier, Nelson, Tebby, Wadsworth, and Wambold, Chapter Six). And we grapple with the tough ethical dilemmas between traditional values and present-day practices.

As Métis, we have responsibilities to our First Nations and Inuit relatives, with whom we have shared these lands (see Hancock, Chapter Seven). We have responsibilities of service that are evident in several chapters in this book—not as the central focus but as mentions that permeate its pages (see Forsythe and Delgado, Chapter One; Fiola, Chapter Five; Forsythe, Chapter Nine; Steele, Chapter Ten; Poitras Pratt and Grant, Chapter Eleven; Delgado, Chapter Thirteen; Tucker, King, Ball, and Gareau, Chapter Fifteen). These can be dedicating one's life to preserving our language, telling our stories, creating spaces for Métis gatherings, community-building, and knowledge sharing, being responsive to the needs of our communities, or simply showing up for each other on date nights. This selflessness runs contrary to the potential monetary benefits or employment opportunities sought by those who self-Indigenize and claim to be Métis for personal gain (see Boyer and Simard Smith, Chapter Four). We are not saying that all Métis people are selfless, but service prioritization is an emergent theme throughout the contributions to this and other Métis volumes. Listen for it as people share their positions and stories.

Other common threads include the importance of food in many contexts and the valuing of arts with respect to representation and education (see Red River Métis Readers, Chapter Two; Supernant, Haines, Mallet Gauthier, Nelson, Tebby, Wadsworth, and Wambold, Chapter Six; Steele, Chapter Ten; Poitras Pratt and Grant, Chapter Eleven; Porter, Chapter Twelve; Delgado, Chapter Thirteen; Porter, Chapter Fourteen; Tucker, King, Ball, and Gareau, Chapter Fifteen). Our modes of expression are as diverse as any, including fiction, mosaic, fiddling, hip-hop, jigging, beading, digital storytelling, opera, poetry, and sex.

We also privilege the stories and contributions of Métis women and queer Métis (see Red River Métis Readers, Chapter Two; Supernant, Haines, Mallet Gauthier, Nelson, Tebby, Wadsworth, and Wambold, Chapter Six; Forsythe, Chapter Nine; Steele, Chapter Ten; Porter, Chapter Twelve; Fowler, Chapter Thirteen; Tucker, King, Ball, and Gareau, Chapter Fifteen). As many chapters show, Métis work can be intergenerational (see Forsythe and Fowler, Chapter One; Leddy, Chapter Three; Fiola, Chapter Five; Forsythe, Chapter Nine; Steele, Chapter Ten; Poitras Pratt and Grant, Chapter Eleven; Porter, Chapter Twelve; Tucker, King, Ball, and Gareau, Chapter Fifteen). Our studies can focus on health in relation to place, traumatic experience, and cultural connection (see Foulds, LaFleur, and Ferguson, Chapter Eight).

This collection has many threads of commonalities and differences. Each author is Métis, and thus so is each chapter. As Métis, we have many teachers and are teachers ourselves. We laugh together and cry together. We can be brutally honest and exposed. We show strength and vulnerability. We unite and recognize each other with respect, love, critique, and generosity. There are no free passes for being Métis. We are accountable to ourselves, our families, our communities, our kin, and our distinct identities as *Métis Coming Together*.

References

Absolon, K. E. (2011). *Kaandossiwin: How we come to know*. Fernwood Publishing.

Absolon, K. E., & Willett, C. (2005). Putting ourselves forward: Location in Aboriginal research. In L. Brown & S. Strega (Eds.), *Research as resistance: Critical, Indigenous, and anti-oppressive approaches* (pp. 97–126). Canadian Scholars Press.

Adese, J., Todd, Z., & Stevenson, S. (2017). Mediating Métis identity: An interview with Jennifer Adese and Zoe Todd. *MediaTropes*, 7(1), 1–25. https://mediatropes.com/index.php/Mediatropes/article/view/29157/21708

Daniels v. Canada (Indian Affairs and Northern Development), 2016 SCC 12, [2016] 1 S.C.R. 99. https://scc-csc.lexum.com/scc-csc/scc-csc/en/item/15858/index.do

Graveline, F. J. (2000). Circle as methodology: Enacting an Aboriginal paradigm. *International Journal of Qualitative Studies in Education*, *13*(4), 361–370. https://doi.org/10.1080/09518390041330

Kovach, M. (2009). *Indigenous methodologies: Characteristics, conversations, and contexts*. University of Toronto Press.

Kovach, M. (2017). Doing Indigenous methodologies. In N. K. Denzin & Y. S. Lincoln (Eds.). *The SAGE handbook of qualitative research* (5th ed.), pp. 383–406. SAGE.

Kovach, M. (2021). *Indigenous methodologies: Characteristics, conversations, and contexts* (2nd ed.). University of Toronto Press.

LaRocque, E. (1975). *Defeathering the Indian*. The Book Society of Canada.

McGregor, D., Restoule, J. P., & Johnston, R. (Eds.). (2018). *Indigenous research: Theories, practices, and relationships*. Canadian Scholars Press.

Moreton-Robinson, A. (2017). Relationality: A key presupposition of an Indigenous social research paradigm. In C. Andersen & J. M. O'Brien (Eds.), *Sources and methods in Indigenous studies* (pp. 69–77). Routledge.

Shore, F. J. (2018). *Threads in the sash: The story of the Métis people*. Pemmican Publications.

Smith, L. Tuhiwai (2012). *Decolonizing methodologies: Research and Indigenous peoples*. Zed Books.

· 1 ·

THE REASON WE GATHER: MÉTIS-SPECIFIC SPACES

Laura Forsythe and Lucy Delgado

Taanshi. We are two Métis women who are also mothers, daughters, sisters, spouses, educators, and researchers, and our academic work aligns with our personal dreams and goals of empowering our community and creating opportunities for celebrating Métis peoples. This article articulates how one such opportunity, the Mawachihitotaak Métis Symposium, came to pass in May 2022 and its resulting impacts on community members who attended, as reported on a post-symposium survey.

We introduce ourselves to position ourselves within our research and adhere to Métis research positionality protocols (e.g., Acoose, 1995; Adese et al., 2017; LaRocque, 1975, 2015). Laura Forsythe d-ishinikaashon. My name is Laura Forsythe. Ma famii kawyesh Roostertown d-oshciwak. My family was from Rooster Town a long time ago. Anosh ma famii Winnipeg wikiwak. Today, my family lives in Winnipeg. Ma Parentii (my ancestors) are Huppe, Ward, Berard, Morin, Lavallee, and Cyr. Niya en Michif. I am Métis from the Red River Settlement and grew up in the heart of the Métis Homeland, like the generations of women before me. My maternal great-grandmother Nora Berard was born in Rooster Town on land known as lot 31, owned by my ancestor Jean Baptiste Berard, and my lineage includes Joseph Huppe, who fought in the Victory of Frog Plain.

Lucy Delgado d-ishinikaashon, Winnipeg d-oschin p dan Winnipeg niwiikin. En Michif niya. I am Lucy Fowler, a two-spirit Métis woman, born and raised in Winnipeg, Manitoba. My family were Sinclairs, Cummings, Prudens, some of whom took scrip in St. Andrews and St. Johns, and I have other family and ancestors from Red River, Oxford House, Norway House, and Sioux Valley and settler ancestors from Ireland and the Orkney Islands. I am an academic and community organizer, with a research and teaching focus on Métis youth identity, Indigenous education, queer theory, and youth cultures.

As we share the names and stories of our families, we pay tribute to the work they did and the lives they led, which allowed us to be here in these academic halls. We also name our ancestors and our homelands to build connections with each other and you, the reader, and invite you to think of your ancestors too.

To understand the significance of the Mawachihitotaak symposium, it is essential to understand the context in which it happened, which we provide by discussing Métis gatherings across the homelands more generally before telling the story of the Mawachihitotaak symposium, sharing the preliminary findings and themes of the post-symposium survey, and finally discussing what we see as the next steps for Métis gatherings across the homeland.

Past Métis Gatherings

Our examination of the history of Métis-specific gatherings in Canada between 1980 and 2022 found 40 such instances. Due to the exclusive nature of many Métis gatherings and shifts in promotion over the past 40 years, there are undoubtedly gaps yet to be filled. Nevertheless, the data collected provide an overview of the offerings of the past. The focus of the 40 Métis-specific gatherings from 1980 to 2022 were of four types: (1) politically driven gatherings offered by either specific Métis governing bodies or the Métis National Council (MNC), (2) culturally focused gatherings intended to educate the wider community and hosted by the Gabriel Dumont Institute (GDI), (3) language gatherings centered on Michif hosted by either the nation or the GDI, and (4) academic conferences.

In the first form, Métis governing bodies—the Manitoba Métis Federation (MMF), Métis Nation Saskatchewan (MNS), Métis Nation of Alberta (MNA), Métis Nation British Columbia (MNBC), and Métis Nation Ontario (MNO)—have held Métis-specific gatherings outside their annual general assemblies. However, the majority were politically driven, with many centered on leadership, self-government, and identity. The gatherings covered a number of topics designed for citizens or members of the governing bodies. All five governing bodies have held youth gatherings centered on the nation's future leadership and designed as an opportunity to educate and consult, such as the MNS-hosted Kishkayta in 2021. There is a long history within the nation of hosting Elder conferences such as the MMF's Past reflects the Present: The Métis Elders' Conference in 1991, documented by Barkwell and Shore (1997). Elder gatherings across the homeland brought Elders together to share stories of Métis ways of being and knowing to inform future negotiations when asserting Métis rights. Prior to the fracturing of the governing bodies in 2021, with the MMF leaving the MNC, gatherings have included policy forums inviting representatives from all five governing bodies and an annual celebration at Batoche, all assertions of Métis rights and the need to preserve Métis ways of being.

Over the past four decades, the GDI has hosted a series of conferences mainly around education and sharing cultural understandings. In 1976, the Association of Métis and Non-Status Indians of Saskatchewan began to dream of a conference, which materialized in 1980 with the first GDI conference. In the early years, these annual conferences were inclusive of all nations, bringing in Métis speakers such as the scholars Rita Bouvier and Sherry Farrell Racette and Yvon Dumont, a former MMF president, while also welcoming First Nation speakers such as Elijah Harper (Oji-Cree politician), Verna Kirkness (Cree scholar), and Winona Wheeler (Cree/Assiniboine/Saulteaux and English/Irish scholar) (GDI, 1991). Attendees in the early years included GDI students and a selective guest list. The themed gatherings featured language revitalization, culture, justice reform, identity, and self-governance. Recently, GDI celebrated the 40th anniversary of its culture conference with an event featuring 42 sessions on a wide range of topics from beading to genealogy and memoir writing. The celebration included scholars, politicians, and community members, with a limited number of the 320 attendees required to purchase a ticket.

In the 1980s, the governing bodies and institutes started to host Michif language conferences and gatherings. The movement started in the MMF with the creation of the Michif Language Committee in 1984 and the Michif Language Conference, featuring 70 delegates from Manitoba, Saskatchewan, Alberta, and North Dakota (Louis Riel Institute, 2023). In 2019, Sakitawak Elders held the 20th Annual Michif Language Festival in Île-à-la-Crosse, Saskatchewan, which featured a celebration with music and speakers and culminated in the signing of a declaration to uphold Métis ways of being by all leaders in attendance. In addition, in the spring of 2023, the GDI held an invite-only National Michif Speakers Gathering to discuss promising practices around language revitalization (GDI, 2023).

There has also been an increase in Métis-specific conferences or symposia in a post-secondary setting over the past decade. For example, the University of Alberta, in partnership with the MNA and Rupertsland Institute, hosted two conferences dealing with Métis-specific content at the post-secondary institutional level: the *Daniels* Conference: In and Beyond Law (2017) and the Métis Land: Rights and Scrip Conference (2019). Both were open to the public and centered in the academy. Scholars nationwide were invited to present their research on Métis history, land claims, scrip, and rights.

During the pandemic, there was a surge in virtual gatherings hosted by the five governing bodies across the homeland, giving institutions a wider audience; geographical location was no longer a barrier to participation, and many events were free. Such gatherings included the MMF's Red River Métis Youth Conference on Identity, the Métis Nation of Saskatchewan's a tayr, la laang pi li rispay—Land, Language and Respect and The Exchange of Western and Traditional Knowledge, and the MNC's Indigenous Protected and Conserved Areas and Métis Guardians.

It is essential to honor the work that has come before, which we have done by highlighting the four types of gatherings that played a role in keeping Métis ways of knowing and Métis understandings of self in community conversations. While these events may have been exclusive due to an attendance requirement of connection or affiliation with the governing bodies and/or institutes, acknowledgment of their role is essential to understanding the inclusive design of the Mawachihitotaak symposium.

Mawachihitotaak: Let's Get Together

Months before the Mawachihitotaak Métis Symposium was even a concept, a group of Métis scholars from across the homeland, called Li Rooñ por kaanatonikeechik (The Circle for Those Who Research), began to meet on Zoom to share ideas, discuss research, and build an academic community for Métis scholars. The 2021 conference season disheartened many Métis scholars in the group with a lack of inclusion of Métis-specific research and low Métis acceptance rates by non-Indigenous conference organizers. Scholarship exploring the lack of Métis-specific research and programming (Binn et al.,

2021; Forsythe, 2023; Kumar et al., 2012; Logan, 2008; Monchalin, 2019; Scott, 2021) has documented this lived experience of Métis scholars and the toll that lack of representation takes. Through visiting in Li Rooñ por kaa-natonikeechik meetings, we decided to create our own academic Métis space. Reaching out to our community kinship ties, 32 Métis thinkers volunteered to create a Métis-centric conference in response to our collective need to see a space celebrating our research and community.

These 32 scholars who came together to bring this symposium to life came from 12 post-secondary institutions across Canada, the Louis Riel Institute, and the Prairies to Woodlands Indigenous Language Revitalization Circle. Those who sat to plan and execute the event ranged from language keepers and community members to undergraduate and graduate students and scholars at various stages in their academic careers. Their names and affiliations at the time of the symposium can be found in the appendix to this chapter.

The structure of the organizing committee differed from similar bodies on which planners had served in the past. Instead of a hierarchy, we decided to call our organizing group the Métis thinkers and approach the planning, fundraising, and organizing collectively. Several Métis thinkers were also planners of "Kwaata-nihtaawakihk—A Hard Birth," an exhibit to be mounted at the Winnipeg Art Gallery in May 2022, and we were able to plan the conference in partnership with the exhibit.

It was essential to many of the Métis thinkers that attendees be able to join and learn without paying exorbitant fees, so funding became very important. Most funding for the conference came from the Métis scholars' own SSHRC or start-up funds, as well as the funds from three Métis Canada Research Chairs. The University of Manitoba Métis University Students Association applied for a student luncheon through the Rising Youth grant, and several of the Métis thinkers received funding from the University of Manitoba Indigenous Initiatives Fund. The combination of these diverse funding sources enabled us to offer the conference at no cost to attendees.

As excitement grew for possibly being together again following the first two years of the pandemic, Elder Verna Demontigny gifted us with the name Mawachihitotaak, meaning "let's get together" in Southern Michif. Momentum grew, and we began to call out to the community for those who would like to share their knowledge. We wanted academics and community members doing important work with and for Métis peoples to feel welcomed in this conference space. An overwhelming number of proposals came to us, and an even more overwhelming number of people wanted to witness the symposium.

We planned panels and workshops with the space at the Winnipeg Art Gallery in mind, but public health concerns changed some of these plans. A few months before the conference, the COVID-19 strain Omicron emerged, and the grandmothers shared that now was not the time to get together in person. While putting aside our dreams of spending time together after so much time apart was challenging, we were thankful for their wisdom and decided to move the conference to a virtual space. We had all been part of several years of virtual gatherings by that point and were able to deploy these experiences in our planning. Being in a virtual space together meant that the flight delays that plagued summer 2022 did not impact conference attendance, and as pandemic numbers spiked again in the days leading up to the conference, we were again thankful to the grandmothers for the wisdom and words that kept us safe.

Mawachihitotaak took place from May 3–6, 2022, and brought together over 2000 attendees from all over Canada and the United States. Registration was open to all at no cost. In the opening keynote, Chris Andersen spoke to a large audience about Métis leadership in the academy. The conference featured 113 Métis scholars, knowledge holders, language speakers, community organizers, writers, art makers, students, and other community leaders who shared their knowledge and engaged in conversation. Sessions ranged from presentations, roundtable discussions, panels, workshops, artist talks, art interventions, film screenings, musical performances, and poetry, spoken word, and literature readings. Maria Campbell closed the conference with storytelling and teachings about walking forward. Many sessions were recorded and available to attendees for 10 days following the conclusion of the conference in an attempt to ensure that those with obligations like jobs or family would still have a chance to learn from Métis scholars and community members.

Themes and Discussion

Following the conference's conclusion, participants were given the link to a survey intended to gauge the impact of the conference, areas that could be improved for the next iteration, and the experiences of those who had attended. Out of over 2000 attendees, we received 126 responses to the survey. When examining the responses to the post-conference survey, three central themes arose: (1) learning, listening, and sharing through a Métis lens, (2) connecting to Métis identity, and (3) strengthening and connecting Métis community.

Many survey respondents explained that they had participated in the symposium out of interest in research and community work that spoke explicitly to Métis experiences and needs. One respondent reported attending to "learn about all the beautiful things Métis people are doing and working on, hearing stories from kin and digging deeper into our history and the ties that keep us woven together." As noted above, there have not been many Métis community gatherings that have been open to the public, and survey respondents were excited to share their knowledge or work and to learn from others. Because of the opportunity to attend the symposium online at no cost, community members and students who might not have been able to pay travel or registration expenses were able to participate. Others were interested in bringing knowledge and research practices from the conference back into their work, whether in academia, government, or the private and third sectors. Respondents also noted the draw of some familiar names in Métis studies—either because of their own educational experiences with those scholars or the significance of their work in the field. Several respondents noted that the array of presenters was a draw and that senior scholars, emerging scholars, and community members were not differentiated in terms of importance. Some had never been selected to present at a conference and felt honored to be accepted onto the program. Several respondents spoke about wanting to "learn more about Métis everything and hear Métis stories" and "craving more authentic first-hand conversation, not a regurgitated history lesson or patriarchal/hierarchical vision of history." Another respondent noted that this conference was the first they had been to that acknowledged the "human-emotional-spiritual side of research and learning" and shared that this made it one of the best conferences they had ever attended.

The second theme that arose in the responses was connecting to Métis identity. This conference was uniquely Métis: the organizing team was entirely Métis, all presenters needed to be either Métis or presenting alongside Métis people, and 82% ($n = 103$) of attendees who responded to the survey were Métis. Many survey respondents shared that attending this symposium was a way to learn and connect to their own identity as Métis people. This learning varied, as some had not previously been connected to a Métis community and were learning things about their people for the first time, and others found their sense of self strengthened, as presentations for one respondent "reinforced so many experiences of what Métis peoplehood looks like and helped me to expand my own understanding." Another respondent spoke about the ways in which and reasons why many Métis people need events like Mawachihitotaak to connect to their own identities, sharing that the active attempt to erase the existence of Métis people by colonial mainstream governments has driven so much of their culture underground and that most Métis doubt their own identities. Especially in the context of ongoing identity appropriation and reactionary identity policing, they may not feel comfortable claiming or inhabiting them. Métis-centered events reveal that familial traits as cultural and help identify and process shared trauma, create and maintain a community of accountability, and foster cultural resurgence.

Several other respondents also noted that their family histories included disconnection from Métis identity and culture and that participating in this conference had helped them learn more about themselves and "reinforced so many experiences of what Métis peoplehood looks like and helped me to expand my own understanding." This multitude of experiences helped dismantle ideas of "not feeling Métis enough" to participate in Métis events, as one participant put it. Being surrounded by other Métis peoples with similar stories of identity and belonging (as was sure to be the case with so many attendees) meant that the symposium participants saw themselves reflected in scholarship and the community.

The third theme among respondents was the strengthening of connections to the Métis community. Many respondents expressed that in their own lives, they often felt isolated from the Métis community and culture for a variety of reasons, including the "diasporic nature of our people" and living away from the homelands, being the only Métis scholars in their areas or their institutions, and not having connections with other Métis peoples. One respondent said, "I am a Métis scholar and feel isolated. I wanted a sense of community to support and to receive support from." Through attending this symposium, respondents felt less isolated, because of feeling more connected to the community (even if virtually), being able to visit, or hearing from and bearing witness to so many others sharing similar experiences. Respondents said that being able to be in community with other Métis people across the diaspora allowed them to "honor who we are as a distinct community" and "learn from one another and deepen together as community." In the context of the academy, where so much of the focus is on Indigenization more broadly, this symposium carved out a space for Métis knowledges, experiences, and realities to be showcased and reflected. If anything, this experience has shown the organizers the strength of the hunger within the community for similar events and reinforced the need to prioritize Métis scholarly spaces.

Conclusion

We conceived a Métis research symposium out of conversations in Li Rooñ por kaa-natonikeechik, the Métis research circle. We had come together in that space to share ideas, obtain feedback, and commiserate and celebrate with other Métis scholars, and it was clear we had the critical mass needed to support both organizing the conference and presenting the panels we had in mind. We knew this work was necessary because a limited number of Métis-specific gathering spaces had been open to the public in the past, and no gatherings that focused on Métis research were open to the public. As Métis scholars, we felt the same yearning for community, camaraderie, and allies in the often isolating world of academia. We asked how to foster a sense of belonging and a sense of worth in academia. Our response to this question was creating this conference as a first step in developing a community of Métis researchers dedicated to working with and for the nation and celebrating one another's work. We look to continue this work—although it is surely a labor of love—for Métis people by creating more Métis-specific opportunities: journals, symposiums, gatherings, workshops, and writing groups. Through this work, we attend to our community members' needs, dreams, and desires and hope to provide opportunities and support for our colleagues today and those coming after us. Building community and prioritizing relationships are central to our culture, and we continue to look to this work to feed the need in the community and in ourselves for reconnection and Métis ways of being.

Appendix

The Métis thinkers who contributed to designing and implementing the Mawachihitotaak Métis Symposium are listed below in alphabetical order, with their affiliations at the time.

> Jennifer Adese, University of Toronto-Mississauga
> Vicki Bouvier, Mount Royal University
> Maria Campbell, University of Saskatchewan
> Shirley Delorme Russell, Louis Riel Institute
> Verna DeMontigny, Prairie to Woodlands Indigenous Language Revitalization Circle
> Chantal Fiola, University of Winnipeg

Lucy Fowler, University of Manitoba
Chelsea Gabel, McMaster University
Mylene Gamache, University of Manitoba
Paul Gareau, University of Alberta
Janice Cindy Gaudet, University of Alberta
Sharon Goulet, University of Manitoba
Nicki Ferland, University of Saskatchewan
Laura Forsythe, University of Winnipeg
Rob Hancock, University of Victoria
Sarah Hourie, University of Manitoba
Kiera Kowalski, University of Winnipeg
Melanie Lalonde, University of Manitoba
Amanda LaVallee, University of the Fraser Valley
Lynn Lavallée, Toronto Metropolitan University
Jennifer Markides, University of Calgary
Cathy Mattes, University of Winnipeg
Victoria May, Concordia University
Alexandra Nychuk, McMaster University
David Parent, University of Manitoba
Jeremy Patzer, University of Manitoba
Brielle Lucille Beaudin Reimer, University of Manitoba
Allyson Stevenson, University of Saskatchewan
Nicole Stonyk, University of Manitoba
Heather Souter, University of Manitoba
Cheryl Troupe, University of Saskatchewan
Angie Tucker, University of Alberta

References

Acoose, J. (1995). *Iskwewakkah' Ki Yaw Ni Wahkomakanak: Neither Indian princesses nor easy squaws*. Women's Press.
Adese, J., Todd, Z., & Stevenson, S. (2017). Mediating Métis identity: An interview with Jennifer Adese and Zoe Todd. *MediaTropes*, 7(1). 1–25. https://mediatropes.com/index.php/Mediatropes/article/view/29157/21708
Barkwell, L. J., & Shore, F. J. (Eds.). (1997). *Past reflects the present: The Métis elders' conference*. Manitoba Métis Federation.
Binn, D., Canada, D., Chenoweth, J., & Neel, L. A. (2021). Pulling together: A guide for researchers, Hitk̓ala. *BCcampus*. https://opentextbc.ca/indigenizationresearchers/

Gabriel Dumont Institute. (1991). *Education and the family.* https://www.metismuseum.ca/media/document.php/12795.Annual%20Cultural%20Conference,%201991,%20overview.pdf

Kumar, M. B., Wesche, S., & McGuire, C. (2012). Trends in Métis-related health research (1980–2009): Identification of research gaps. *Canadian Journal of Public Health, 103*(1), 23–28. https://doi.org/10.1007/BF03404064

LaRocque, E. (1975). *Defeathering the Indian.* The Book Society of Canada.

LaRocque, E. (2015). Foreword: Resist no longer: Reflections on resistance writing and teaching. In E. Coburn (Ed.), *More will sing their way to freedom: Indigenous resistance and resurgence* (pp. 5–23). Fernwood Publishing.

Logan, T. (2008). Métis scholarship in the 21st century: Life on the periphery. In K. Knopf (Ed.). *Aboriginal Canada revisited* (pp. 88–99). University of Ottawa Press.

Louis Riel Institute (2023). Michif Language Conference. https://www.lriarchives.ca/collection/michif-language-conference-1985

Monchalin, R. (2019). *Digging up the medicines: Urban Métis women's identity and experiences with health and social services in Toronto, Ontario* [Doctoral dissertation, University of Toronto]. https://hdl.handle.net/1807/97587

Scott, B. (2021). Métis women's experiences in Canadian higher education. *Genealogy, 5*(2), Article 49. https://doi.org/10.3390/genealogy5020049

· 2 ·

RED RIVER READERS IN MULTIVOCAL FLUX: ACROSS, BETWEEN, AND BEYOND TRADITIONAL DISCIPLINARY APPROACHES TO MÉTIS STUDIES

Red River Readers

We write this piece as a Red River Métis collective composed of five readers whose individual stories are conveyed through critical engagement with three works of contemporary Métis life writing: Maria Campbell's *Halfbreed* (2019), Marilyn Dumont's *A Really Good Brown Girl* ([1996], 2015), and Katherine Vermette's *The Strangers* (2021). As an assemblage of Indigenous Studies students and professors at the University of Manitoba, we have come to know one another over the past three years and in varying combinations as co-learners and colleagues in shared classrooms and university spaces. In our capacity as a collective, we presented our ideas as a panel during the Mawachihitotaak Métis Symposium, where we assessed how Campbell, Dumont, and Vermette, as agents of Métis storywork (Archibald, 2008), incited us to conceptualize Métis life writing as the basis of theory. We were interested in how Métis studies produces itself in and beyond the classroom, and how present and future Métis studies practitioners continue to center Métis historic and contemporary immediacies. In returning to Gaudry and Hancock's (2012) paper on decolonizing Métis pedagogies a decade later, our Mawachihitotaak panel was also prompted to ask whose and what places are being centered in Métis studies co-learning spaces. Gaudry and Hancock (2012) focus specifically on the decolonial potential of Métis students sharing classroom space and discussing works by Métis scholars while considering the relationships between learners and the lands on which they live. Yet, at the time both Gaudry and Hancock were writing from the context of Victoria, British Columbia, a place located outside the homeland of the Métis nation. Our initial roundtable discussion sought to consider similar questions and perspectives in the context of living and learning in the Red River Valley, the birthplace of the Métis nation, and the place we each call home. While we recognize that we are engaging with Métis life writings across the Métis homeland, each writer engages with the specificity of place in ways which reflect her own lived understandings of Métis mobilities in the later twentieth century and in the present. Rather than reifying a Red River-centric perspective, we amplify ways in which place-based narratives and multiplicities engage in multivocal conversation with each other.

Since at least 1975, contemporary Métis scholars have discussed the issue of misrepresentation as it pertains to Indigenous peoples in Canada broadly and to the Métis on the North American prairies more specifically. In their respective books, Emma LaRocque (1975) and Howard Adams (1975) both deconstruct how Métis and other Indigenous peoples come to misrecognize themselves through dominant misrepresentations of who they are. LaRocque (1975) distinguishes between culture, which evolves, and historic heritage, whose conflation has led to misrepresentations where Métis practices are static and "frozen" in the past (pp. 8, 13). The ossification of culture and heritage occurs for Adams (1975) when Métis and other Indigenous peoples are relegated to this static point in time, which then functions as a "traditional" or "authentic" matrix through which Métis come to be assessed and to assess themselves (p. 36). Since then, we have seen Métis scholars interrogate both the misrepresentations of the Métis in history and literature, along with our continued misrecognition in fields where social scientific data are used to define Métis, as Chris Andersen and others have established following the *Powley* decision.

Métis studies scholars are no longer stuck in the continued response and feedback loop of negotiating who we are based on who we are not: "mixed" (Adese & Andersen, 2021). All three works discussed at our panel speak to their authors' vulnerabilities and the ethics of engagement by "reasserting control over the representation of Métis people through autobiography, poetry, and fiction" (Gaudry & Hancock, 2012, p. 9). Vermette, Dumont, and Campbell place their Métis protagonists and speakers in positions of creation, as they are informed by and inform reproductions of Métis culture and epistemologies in their specific contexts. This idea deconstructs the misconception that culture or learning can only take place in fixed settings. Instead, characters in everyday circumstances bring their ingenuity to the forefront as they stay connected to place and maintain their relations to who they are. As such, these works help us locate what it means to be Métis in different spatial and temporal contexts in a way that challenges the misrepresentations of Métis in court decisions or some secondary research that produce racialized understandings of Métis identity and static representations of Métis culture.

We begin our discussion by illustrating how Métis life writings are indicative of what Chris Andersen has described as Indigenous *density*. Métis biopower is produced through these life writings specifically because they dare to focus on the presence and persistence of Métis life, as opposed to its absence. Following our discussion of the density of Métis life writings, we then conspire to produce a relational Indigenous existentialism that combines both the âcimowina (factual stories) and âcimisowina (autobiographical stories) of Campbell, Dumont, and Vermette, interwoven with our own. In doing so, we amplify not simply the density of the authors with whom we've engaged but also the density present among ourselves and the relations that we have and that continue to allow us to exist and persist in the present, regardless of whether we are "resistant" or "resilient" for white gazes. Moreton-Robinson (2021) writes that whiteness "defines itself by what it is not" (p. 312): it comes into being through the demarcation of difference inasmuch as racialization occurs through an insistent drive for cultural difference that reinforces entrapment within systems of white possession (Moreton-Robinson, 2015, 2016). Drawing from Andersen (2009), Moreton-Robinson (2016) argues that "the critique of whiteness must be a central element in any Indigenous studies discipline, a proposition that provides direction for Indigenous scholars to unpack the complexity of the relationship between racialized knowledge and the production of cultural density" (p. 104). Furthermore, as we demonstrate through the writings of Vermette, Campbell, and Dumont and through our own reflections, Métis experiences of whiteness demonstrate how "white identity has cultural and social purchase, and as a possession it enhances one's life chances as configured through the logic of capital" (Moreton-Robinson, 2015, p. xix). As Métis writers show, such an analysis can be woven throughout Métis life writings in multifaceted ways, such that Métis come to both imagine the desirability of whiteness while also demarcating for themselves the ways in which it has come to (re)shape daily life.

Métis Density Through Life Writing: "Nothing Less Than the Sum of Our Life Writings"

In this chapter, we echo Andersen's (2014) suggestion that narratives of dispossession that recenter the Red River Resistance and the Battle of Batoche continually emphasize Métis loss and deficit. How do we overcome a hegemonic Indigenous Studies discourse that continues to redefine Métis authenticity through experiences of dispossession and deficit? What stories are buried through consistent calls for resurgence, when such stories require the disavowal of the density and endurance of our relatives, of the continuity of our Indigeneity, and of our relations to place and to one another?

Even as loss permeates these hegemonic narratives, we suggest that these dominant stories are also ones of Métis density. Drawing on the theoretical richness of Black Studies historian Robin Kelly, Chris Andersen importantly argues in 2009 that Indigenous scholars, including Métis, not only must move beyond studying solely how they are "different" from whitestream institutions and society but also consider how we have theorized our own engagements with such institutions and become experts of normalizing forms of whiteness. *Density requires considering how Indigenous persons come to experience white systems differently and differentially, as specific sites of knowledge production about whiteness are constituted through these intersections.* Our collective engagements here extend Andersen's (2014) call to also consider thinking beyond deficit and toward Métis density, in order to conceptualize "our modernity" as Métis (p. 621).

In "More Than the Sum of Our Rebellions" (2014), Chris Andersen describes one of the challenges facing scholars of the Métis experience:

> Much of the existing discussion pertaining to everyday-life kinds of issues comes not from scholarly research but rather in the context of personal narrative and reminiscence in the form of biographies and autobiographies of Métis people and communities or government-sponsored socio-economic surveys. While fascinating in their own right, neither of these literatures offers much in the way of analysis that links subjective experiences to structural contexts and the changing political economies of the region and era (pp. 628–629).

Life writings, however, are more than just fascinating biographical accounts; they are also sites of generative critique and factual accountings of institutions as they have come to "produce Indigeneity" (Hokowhitu, 2013). In response to Andersen, we argue that Campbell, Dumont, and Vermette illustrate how structural contexts work upon their characters and that they do so in ways that demonstrate "felt knowledge" of whiteness (Million, 2009). They do this through illustrating how institutional structures come to be bodily and psychically inscribed in the twentieth and twenty-first centuries, thus forming sites of embodied knowledges which then reshape Indigenous constructions of whiteness and knowledge of institutions that buoy its dominance. Through these writings, Vermette, Campbell, and Dumont demonstrate an expertise in whiteness as it has come to matter to them.

Throughout this piece, we deliberately position ourselves as Métis without emphasizing imagined or shared lived experiences, without singularizing one nationalist narrative, without limning one coherent narrative voice. To emphasize the density of this reading group and our engagements across genres and styles, we work to position ourselves in relation to these dense life narratives rather than in efforts to legitimate ourselves through dominant narratives of dispossession (scrip), poverty, significant political events, national historic sites, and family names. Campbell, Dumont, and Vermette challenge institutional accountings of Métis people that often misrecognize histories by refocusing their stories as knowers of whiteness. Insofar as our voices are neither unified nor blended, this fraught "we" occasionally gives way to an indistinct "I."

While making clear the distinction between difference and density, Campbell's *Halfbreed* allows me to intimately understand and contextualize the generation of my grandmother through Maria's choices and experiences, which were affected by the gaze of whiteness, as reflected in narratives of land dispossession, poverty, and moving to Vancouver's city center. Although their stories are situated in different parts of the Métis homeland and beyond, Campbell's writing provides an understanding of the specific challenges and perils Métis women in my grandmother's generation faced, thus allowing a vicarious connection to my own Métis identity. Cheechum warns Campbell in *Halfbreed* (2019) that "the white man saw that [the desire for whiteness] was a more powerful weapon than anything else with which to beat the Halfbreeds, and he used it and still does today. Already they are using it on you. They try to make you hate your people" (p. 52). Cheechum later metaphorically explains that people wear blankets in their own way to cover their shame and that one day, "people would throw them away and the whole world would change" (Campbell, 2019, p. 163). The juxtaposition of the blanket worn by Métis who feel they need to cover up who they are and those who wear it because they are not "Métis enough" produces further planes of misrecognition amongst our own. Perhaps the varied ways in which we wear our blankets are in fact pointing toward revealing the complexity of differences shared in and through our collective density. While Cheechum reminds Maria, "You'll find yourself, and you'll find brothers and sisters," Campbell (2019) goes on to recognize that, by finding her "brothers and sisters, all over the country, [she] no longer need[s her] blanket to survive" (p. 189).

The Break from the Colonial Dialectic

These texts position and engage representations of and experiences with whiteness through structures of surveillance by society more generally. In each of the texts, the authors describe instances of heightened surveillance of the everyday lives of Métis people that are accessible to readers. They speak to the shared complexities of intergenerational and place-based resistance to surveillance by acknowledging these structures and their effects on Métis identity. The perception of Métis as defined by being othered or through categorizing difference inform the authors' internalization of whiteness and its apparent dangers. Campbell (2019) describes her experiences with shame and hatred of being Métis when one of the girls from her school asks if Sophie—a visibly Halfbreed woman who accompanied her to a dance—was her mother, to which Campbell replies, "'That old, ugly Indian?'" Upon noticing the rejection on Sophie's face, she recalls her Cheechum saying, "'They make you hate what you are'" (p. 103). Campbell's attempts to distance herself from her Métis identity and community are demonstrative of the choices Métis women made to hide their connectedness to people and places in attempts to appear white. Dumont (2015) shares similar experiences when her brother's white fiancée "lathered, scrubbed, shampooed, exfoliated, medicated, pedicured, manicured, rubbed down and moisturized" her, almost as if to disguise her Métis appearance (p. 29). Dumont tries to become invisible to seem adept at deflecting feelings of shame and disappointment. Vermette's description of Margaret Stranger, Elsie's mother and grandmother to Elsie's children, frames sentiments of shame while emphasizing her associated anger and hatred. When her partner was breaking up with her, she became cognizant of not being good enough for any white man. As she writes, "this was the moment she chose to hear it all and know it, accept it. This was the moment she chose to know that no matter how many manicures, permanents, and good clothes she had, she still had never passed enough" (Vermette, 2021, p. 253).

In all three of these accounts, Métis women have noticed, been made aware of, and directly experienced being observed by white people. Each in her own way, they internalized these feelings of hatred and shame. Campbell (2019) describes this process powerfully when sharing the pride and happiness felt by Métis families "until [they] drove into town, then everyone became quiet and looked different. The men walked in front, looking straight ahead, their wives behind, and, [she] can never forget this, they had their heads down and never looked up" (p. 37). The systems of surveillance and its normalization through everyday experiences alter how Métis look at themselves and their communities. We tend to present ourselves in a manner that will not provoke Canadians and their perception of us, and in so doing, we distance ourselves from our communities, families, places and areas not created for us. These authors speak back to these internalized deficits through their own experiences of being rendered deficient, something many of our relatives have surely done in efforts to evade observation and their becoming the object of the white gaze.

When Campbell was growing up, Métis people were perceived as poor, uneducated, and dirty by white families. They withdrew themselves from these communities while simultaneously facing encroachment through urban expansion and federal conservation efforts that criminalized Métis hunting practices. In one example, structures of surveillance shaped Campbell's life as she navigated the welfare office. Her friend Marion advised that she dress the part to receive federal money; she had to embrace the Métis authenticity that was placed onto Métis people by white settlers. She had to look poor. As she recounted, "I went to the Office in a ten-year-old threadbare red coat, with old boots and a scarf. I looked like a Whitefish Lake squaw, and that's exactly what the social worker thought" (Campbell, 2019, p. 155). Similarly, Dumont (2015) shares the density of Métis identity through her encounters of displacement, apologetically identifying as Métis, measuring authenticity temporally, and structuring language. Dumont (2015) as she asserts, "the Great White Way / has measured, judged and assessed me / all my life / [...] one wrong sound and you're shelved in the Native Literature section / resistance writing / a mad Indian / unpredictable / on the war path / [...] the Great White Way could silence us all / if we let it" (p. 73). Her familiarity with the boundaries she must exist in to comply with what she refers to as "the Great White Way" speaks to the multifaceted strategies that Métis people have to employ to navigate structures of surveillance. Vermette (2016) writes about surveillance accessibly as Phoenix's story takes place in the Winnipeg's

Remand Centre, a jail for those awaiting trial. Her experiences with surveillance quite literally take place inside an institution designed and built to survey. Moreover, Phoenix's mother, Elsie, speaks briefly to surveillance through perception. In one account, "Elsie wipes the tears. Looks around but no one notices. No one is paying attention to the strung-out woman on a park bench. She should know that by now. Know how invisible she is. She is" (Vermette, 2016, p. 44). In another, "She crosses the street, trying not to stumble. Doesn't want the people in cars to see her stumble" (Vermette, 2016, p. 50). In both these excerpts, Vermette speaks to the power of surveillance and how it can diminish our perceptions of self over time.

Our authenticity as Métis people is too often constructed as something negative and debilitating that fails to recognize the strengths and endurances of Métis people, and more specifically Métis women. In their related experiences of navigating systems of surveillance, Campbell, Dumont, and Vermette reveal whiteness as hyper-visible (Moreton-Robinson, 2015, p. xiii) and hyper-affective, both to those on whom it comes to bear and to those whom it denies. Their awareness of the dangers and harms of everyday surveillance and their capacities to articulate their vulnerabilities demonstrate their existential persistence. Their expression of connectedness and the importance of recognizing cyclical harm serve as strategies that prevent them from succumbing to it, so their works are crucial to Métis Studies as they share their insecurities about and yet pride in embracing their Métis immediacies.

Toward a Métis Existentialism

> Indigenous existentialism underscores the importance of the lived experience of Indigenous peoples; it moves beyond ressentiment and the focus on "decolonizing the mind" to one of choice and responsibility lost at the juncture of the primitive indigene/civilized European binary, lost when Indigenous peoples became "victims" of colonization. Indigenous existentialism implores Indigenous peoples to move beyond victimhood to reclaim choice and responsibility within their lived experiences. (Hokowhitu, 2013, p. 363).

There is an existentialist current that runs throughout the writings of Vermette, Campbell, and Dumont. During the 2020 season of CBC's Canada Reads, *From the Ashes*, a memoir by Michif scholar and writer Jesse Thistle, was among the candidate books (2022). However, the reception that it was given by judges, including Indigenous judges, derided his account of his experiences as "trauma porn" and a well-worn story through which Canadians have come to know Indigenous peoples in Canada. However, these analyses came to reveal not so much the accuracy of the charges but rather the limiting frameworks through which non-academic and everyday Indigenous people in Canada have come to misrecognize the value of Indigenous density and endurance in our historical present. That is, when read as simply an "Indigenous" account in Canada and extrapolated from the kinscapes of Métis literature that reaffirmed Thistle's experiences and positions, the reduction of his story to a stereotype can easily be analyzed as representative of a kind contemporary Indigenous subjectivity that seeks to contribute to the breadth of density amongst the diversity of Indigenous peoples and nations and how such stories are reflective of what Deanna Reder (2022) and others have theorized as âcimowina or âcimisowina—storying through the sharing of personal experiences.

When âcimowina are read in conversation with each other, however, we are provided with a dynamic space where the confluence of Métis stories come to produce a kind of relational existentialism that demonstrates the historical immediacies of Métis literatures and the excesses that may be too traumatic, messy, or painful to include in a higher level rendering of Métis historiography. That is, through the production of Métis memoirs we are provided with a variety of accounts.

The historical work that Katherena Vermette's *The Break* and *The Strangers* does is to show that narratives about systems of violence need not be the stories that come to define us, even if they may come to reaffirm experiences of such systems. Instead, Vermette illustrates countless examples of what Andersen (2009), in drawing from Moreton-Robinson (2021), has considered density and, specifically, how Indigenous subjectivities are particularly situated to possess a level of expertise regarding whiteness as a social fact of Indigenous existence.

Through the voices of Phoenix, Cedar-Sage, Elsie, and Margaret, the reader is reminded of the finitude of the systems of social control: the child welfare system, prisons, healthcare, and policing,[ii] among others, that have come to be systems about which Métis and other Indigenous peoples in Winnipeg require a specific knowledge set because such systems have come to know Indigeneity in ways that are unrecognizable in the kinds of internal understandings of how Métis families and communities have come to know themselves. That is, Phoenix, Cedar-Sage, Elsie, and Margaret illustrate their own kinds of situated expertise on how *whiteness* has come to shape the limitations and possibilities of their own existences.

> 'Everyone is the way they are for a reason.' She reached for her lighter and her pack of players. A sign that it was time for another rehashing of old memories that contributed to explaining to me how we were made and how we came to be in that moment in time. Stories not of grandeur, but stories of how the world works for Métis women trying to work the world in carceral spaces that can only value them for how hard they worked. Work was never simply the exchange of time, but also the input of creativity, of expression, and of transmissions of knowing.

Vermette, Dumont, and Campbell Write about Experience(s) of Whiteness, and You Should Too

Life stories are unique in their ability to use literary devices to convey specific meanings. The motif of whiteness across all three texts brings readers into tune with their positionality. Maria Campbell's confrontations with white social workers brought me closer to the experiences of my Métis great-grandmother, who lived in the white-dominant community of Starbuck, Manitoba, where the pressures of whiteness with respect to childcare remind readers of the unique position Métis women exercised during the twentieth century and how their density as Métis people allowed them to cope (Campbell, 2019, pp. 122–124). After a visit from relief workers threatening to take action on Campbell's siblings, Campbell (2019) makes a strategic choice to marry a white man who can provide for her and her siblings and to move away from her community to live in Vancouver: "I could tell by his expensive clothes and new car that he could afford to keep us all" (p. 123). Campbell's experiences with whiteness through social services and selectively choosing a marriage partner contextualizes the choices the Métis women in my family had to make to provide security for their children. Instead of feeling that marrying a white man and leaving one's family's community take away from the "Métisness" of our women, Campbell's text shows us that these choices stemming from interactions with whiteness have often come *as a result* of being a Métis woman in the twentieth century and demonstrates how those interactions reflect our density as it persists to this day.

Marilyn Dumont also makes use of the motif of whiteness in "The White Judges," a piece that resonated with my own experiences with whiteness. In exploring the various ways that her family felt the gaze of whiteness in their community, Dumont (2015) describes how she and her siblings "waited till the cardboard boxes / were anonymously dropped at our door, spilling with clothes / waited till we ran swiftly away from the windows and doors / to the farthest room for fear of being seen" (p. 25). Those of us Métis who grew up in poverty may understand Dumont's conflicting feelings about receiving charity in "The White Judges" as common when Dumont attempts to escape the pity and feelings of shame by staying out of sight and in experiencing the inevitability of such engagements with whiteness. Similarly, when the high school I attended in a wealthy, white-dominant neighborhood did food collection drives, I would be the student receiving the cardboard box of food that the largely white students donated. While interactions with whiteness through charity can have connotations of pity and stimulate sentiments of shame, for Dumont (2015), "a box transformed now / into the Sears catalogue" over which she and her siblings shared excitement (p. 26). Dumont demonstrates the density of Métis youth in their ability to come together to overcome shame and find resourcefulness through their relations with whiteness. As a Métis reader, I also felt I was not isolated in my experiences with whiteness and that the ability to contend with and subvert the feelings of shame those interactions can produce is an aspect of Métis density that speaks to our collective intelligibility of grappling with the white gaze that has allowed us to endure.

Vermette (2021) use of whiteness in *The Strangers* also speaks to Métis density. In a scene where Cedar, one of the Métis characters with a history of being in the care of family services, seeks to connect with her biological mother, the white stepmother with whom she now lives responds by saying, "I don't know if I'm comfortable with that" (p. 154). Cedar's knowledge of whiteness shines through the prose, predicting how the stepmother will go on to discuss the reasons why Cedar seeing her biological mother makes her uncomfortable: "I look at her, a little longer than I should. Don't have to ask, she'll tell me anyway" (p. 154). Cedar's confrontation with whiteness in this scene is representative of the knowledge she has embodied as a Métis person and is a way of knowing that is specific to our density as Métis people. I felt this scene demonstrated many of my own experiences with whiteness; while I was in care, white foster parents, counsellors, and social workers also warned against connecting with my biological family. Learning from each of these encounters, I began to approach these conversations in a way that demonstrated my understanding of what whiteness expects of me while living up to my own desires for myself. In this sense, the life story Vermette has crafted brings readers closer to the density of Métis people in our ability to know whiteness and navigate our interactions accordingly so that we can maintain relations and persist as Métis people. It is precisely through our ability to persevere that authors demonstrate the various means of maintaining relations to place and others in the everyday, which speaks to our density as Métis people.

White Ideals of Success

Maria Campbell (2019) writes of Métis encampments with "ten or more families in a long caravan" (p. 35) near the closest town that they would visit during the summers of her youth: "One day we were visited by a committee of indignant townspeople, among them an Indian dressed in a suit, who told us to leave" (p. 39). Another Indigenous man in a suit, also functioning as a kind of colonial placeholder, reappears decades later during a Native activities meeting Campbell attends in Calgary shortly after determining to leave Vancouver once and for all: "The people at those meetings reminded me of that Indian man in a suit who had come to our camp with a delegation of townspeople long ago. They seemed to me to be second-hand suits, whose owners were desperately trying to fit in, but never quite succeeding" (2019, p. 158). Campbell's "mental block about Indians in suits" (p. 171) bespeaks the danger she associates with white markers of approximation. When she later returns home to the Spring River settlement, she once again comes across cross Smoky, who eventually admits to living with a white woman and her sister despite never himself marrying: "You remember how white people used to hate us? Well now they have halfbreed grandchildren all over now"; "Hell," he adds, "some of us are lucky enough to have a white woman to make us feel like we've moved up" (pp. 178–179).

Chris Andersen (2009) suggests that efforts to frame white settler colonialism as wholly repressive rather than simultaneously productive avoids this issue of "how the cultural power of nation-states do not merely oppress but seduce as well" (p. 85). In a reminiscent haze, Campbell writes of relaying to Cheechum, with youthful and "driving ambition," the dream that her brothers and sisters might someday "each have a toothbrush and they'll brush their teeth every day and we'll have a bowl of fruit on the table all the time and (. . .) they'll be able to do anything they want and go anywhere" (2019, p. 138). If Campbell at one moment cedes to such "white ideals of success" (p. 138), she also cautions that "when followed blindly [these dreams] can lead to the disintegration of one's soul" (p. 137).

The allure of white capital commodities and ambitions eventually hardens Margaret, the estranged grandmother in Katherena Vermette's *The Strangers* (2021). At age 14, "She'd walk to Main Street and hitchhike downtown" where she would frequent "dance halls and jazz clubs" whenever she could "pass for older, pass for whiter. The odd time she got turned away, pointed to the more friendly Indian bars, but she had no interest in those. She wanted to dress up and see the pretty people. Those who had a bit of money and owned everything she didn't" (p. 66). Despite Margaret excelling in high school, her teachers would repeatedly dissuade her from attending one of "those old universities" out east (p. 67) and reorient her toward settling on a teaching certificate, which "for a halfbreed was incredible enough, but Margaret had no interest in teaching. She wanted a job where she had to wear the most expensive suits from Eaton's" (p. 67). The desire for the most expensive items, not the "patched clothes" in Dumont's "Blue Ribbon Children" (2015, p. 48), reminds me of my grandmother, who carefully sewed each of her family members' ensembles. A matter of pride and thrift, her careful attention and precision ensured that all three of her daughters and her son were perfectly crisp, as if each had been freshly steam-pressed out of an Eaton's catalogue. My mother later conceded that while aimlessly living for several months in Winnipeg during the mid-1960s, she received a call from my grandmother, who decreed that she was to interview for a teaching position in Ste. Anne. It occurred to me later that my mother may have exacted so much from my sister and me to ensure that we would never doubt either our gifts or our places.

In "The Devil's Language," Dumont (2015) writes that "The Great White Way/ has measured, judged and assessed me all my life/ by its/ lily-white words/ its picket-fence sentences/ and manicured paragraphs" (p. 73). The constant threat of affirming white disciplinary expectations, in writing and in life, dispels a larger concern about the ways in which Métis grapple intergenerationally with assuming their own sense of place. As a young woman, Margaret is moved to physically assault her boyfriend Jacob after she discloses to him her pregnancy, only to have him dismiss any dream of a wedding and reveal to her his own racist predisposition. If at once quietly branded "a mad Indian/ unpredictable/on the war path" (Dumont, 2015, p. 73), the charges following Margaret's physical assault are stayed on the condition that she withdraws from her legal studies and consents to never practice law. Margaret's lawyer insists that this outcome is "the best you can hope for" (Vermette, 2021, p. 257). Both Margaret's grandchildren, Phoenix and Cedar-Sage, are reminded at various times in their lives not to get their hopes up (pp. 214, 218, 219). Yet Vermette's book closes with Cedar-Sage setting herself up in her university dorm in a way that defies colonial prescriptions and places her academic aspirations well within reach: "When everything has a place, clothes in the closet, books on the shelf, all my stuff in a caddy, I look around the room and smile" (p. 332).

(W)riting Métis Worlds

In *Talkin' up to the White Woman*, Aileen Moreton-Robinson (2021) eloquently argues that life writing is theory:

> The term "life writings" has been used because the Indigenous women's texts that have been analysed do not fit the usual strict chronological narrative of autobiography, and they are the product of collaborative lives. In these life writings experience is fundamentally social and relational, not something ascribed separately within the individual. Indigenous women's life writings are based on the collective memories of inter-generational relationships between predominantly Indigenous women, extended families and communities. (p. 35)

The power of life writing is such that it transmits Métis density so clearly that readers are brought into story as a learning experience. Because of life stories' capacity to draw us closer to Métis density, they remain an important asset in Métis studies for combatting racializing and misrepresentative understandings of Métis like those produced in the *Powley* and *Daniels* court decisions.[iii] The undercurrents of legibility that span the lives portrayed in Campbell, Vermette, and Dumont are circumstantial and situated. What we have come to recognize in their writing may not be what Canadians, other Indigenous people, or other Métis for that matter may find. Where some may see poverty, destitution, or "trauma porn," we have come to see reasons for why their worlds and our worlds have come to be how they are. To be sure, these texts are more than the sum of their experiences of whiteness as they have contributed, and continue to contribute, to the present cultural life of the Métis people.

References

Adams, H. (1975). *Prison of grass: Canada from the native point of view*. Vol. 1: New Press.

Adese, J., & Andersen, C. (2021). *A people and a nation: New directions in contemporary Métis studies*. UBC Press.

Andersen, C. (2009). Critical Indigenous studies: From difference to density. *Cultural Studies Review*, 15(2), 80–100. https://epress.lib.uts.edu.au/journals/index.php/csrj/article/view/2039

Andersen, C. (2014). More than the sum of our rebellions: Métis histories beyond Batoche. *Ethnohistory* 61(4), 619–633. https://doi.org/10.1215/00141801-2717795

Archibald, J. (2008, July 21). *Indigenous storywork: Educating the heart, mind, body, and spirit.* UBC Press.

Canadian Broadcasting Corporation. (2020). *George Canyon and Kaniehtiio Horn Discuss 'trauma porn' and portrayals of Indigeneity in literature.* https://www.cbc.ca/books/canadareads/george-canyon-and-kaniehtiio-horn-discuss-trauma-porn-and-portrayals-of-indigeneity-in-literature-1.5656239

Campbell, M. (2019). *Halfbreed.* Penguin Random House

Dumont, M. (1996). *A really good brown girl.* Brick Books.

Gaudry, A., & Hancock, R. L. A. (2012). Decolonizing Métis pedagogies in post-secondary settings. *Canadian Journal of Native Education*, 35(1). https://doi.org/10.14288/cjne.v35i1.196541

Hokowhitu, B. (2009). Indigenous existentialism and the body. *Cultural Studies Review*, 15(2), 101–118. https://epress.lib.uts.edu.au/journals/index.php/csrj/article/view/2040

Hokowhitu, B. (2010a). A genealogy of indigenous resistance. In B. Hokowhitu (Ed.), *Indigenous Identity and Resistance: Researching the Diversity of Knowledge* (pp. XXX–XXX). Otago University Press.

Hokowhitu, B. (Ed.). (2010b). *Indigenous identity and resistance: Researching the diversity of knowledge.* Otago University Press.

Hokowhitu, B. (2013). Producing indigeneity. In E. Peters & C. Andersen (Eds.), *Indigenous in the city: Contemporary identities and cultural innovation* (pp. 354–376). UBC Press.

LaRocque, E. (1975). *Defeathering the Indian.* Book Society of Canada.

Million, D. (2009). Felt theory: An Indigenous feminist approach to affect and history. *Wicazo Sa Review*, 24(2), 53–76.

Moreton-Robinson, A. (2015). *The white possessive: Property, power, and Indigenous sovereignty.* University of Minnesota Press.

Moreton-Robinson, A. (2021). *Talkin'up to the white woman: Indigenous women and feminism.* University of Minnesota Press.

Reder, D. (2022). *Autobiography as Indigenous intellectual tradition: Cree and Métis Âcimisowina.* Wilfrid Laurier University Press.

Thistle, J. (2019). *From the ashes: My story of being Métis, homeless, and finding my way.* Simon & Schuster.

Vermette, K. (2016). *The break.* Anansi Press.

Vermette, K. (2021). *The strangers.* Penguin.

· 3 ·

THE POWER OF DANCING IN TWO WORLDS: FINDING A FIT FOR MÉTIS IDENTITIES IN ACADEMIA

Shannon Leddy

"You don't have to say you are half Métis. You are just Métis." I needed these words. My Uncle, Dan Kane, came to visit me in Vancouver just before Christmas in 2021, and asked to sit in on the last session of the Indigenous Education course I teach in the Faculty of Education at UBC. In introducing him, I spoke about being half-Métis and shared that Uncle Dan was from that side of the family. Later, as I drove him to meet with his daughter, my cousin, he spoke those words to me ... and I could have cried from relief. I didn't grow up with my Métis relatives and despite knowing that I was some kind of Indigenous, it wasn't until I was 31 that I knew which nation I could claim and could claim me. And although that knowledge gave me the drive to pursue a career as an Indigenous educator, that early lack of grounding has always left me feeling a bit like an imposter, despite what my spirit has insisted is my calling.

Now, I can share with confidence and certainty that my father was Patrick Kane, whose father, John Kane, was the son of Mabel Monkman, from St. Louis, Saskatchewan. We are Métis with ancestors who came from St. Paul's Parish in the Red River Valley of Manitoba. All of this is important in following protocol where I now live. I did not grow up introducing myself in this way, and the words still come awkwardly sometimes, but it is how I have learned from our West Coast relations to own and share my place in the world.

Learning to Dance

In this chapter, I explore the complex landscape of navigating Métis identity in an institution of higher learning, where we are still often seen as having hybrid identities or simply not being Indigenous enough. This *less-than* lens can have significant impacts on opportunities and career trajectories in the academy and, worse, can leave Métis scholars in the position of having to defend their Indigenous identities, especially in the light of several recent and very public pretendian revelations in Canada (Cyca, 2022). In this era of truth telling, identity politics, and the notion of post-truth, it is sometimes hard to catch the rhythm of the dance we are in, and we can find ourselves stumbling about uncertainly or simply standing still near the wall, waiting to be noticed and asked. But academia is a hard enough gig to navigate without all this dancing too.

I want to look at Métis identity as a power position, highlighting the ontological and epistemological flexibility that dancing between two worlds allows. In my experience, raised by a white mother but with clear Indigenous roots and ample opportunity to learn from Indigenous friends and community members as I was growing up in Saskatoon, the ability to navigate both worlds has been an enormous advantage in teaching and learning at every level. It has helped me to dance in and between two worlds and create bridges between different ways of knowing and being. Drawing on both personal experience and some current scholarship, I seek to create with this chapter an opportunity to nurture the empowerment of Métis scholars who may also be struggling with how they fit into the academy. Tâwâw—there is room for you here.

Dancing with the Darkside

Even now, as a newly tenured scholar, I remain very conscious of the limitations of my own cultural learning and of my identity. This is especially true in a post-secondary setting and most particularly when I am working with other Indigenous faculty and students. I did not grow up on a reservation, and I do not speak Michif. I am a Nehiyawan (Cree) language learner because that is the closest I can get to learning Michif in Vancouver. I do not know all the rules that apply to status and tuition at post-secondary institutions, and I teach on the homeland of the Musqueam, so I am also a guest in the place I have chosen to live.

But the academy puts limits on me based on my identity too. I have been passed over for opportunities and excluded from receiving credit for work I have done for my institution. At the same time, I am in constant demand as an Indigenous representative on hiring committees, advisory boards, and working groups, where my outspoken nature has earned me a reputation as a strong Indigenous advocate who can be relied upon to keep beating the same drum and to work in relationally ethical ways. And I know that this is expected of me. I am always not enough for some, dancing too slow, even as I dance too much and too fast for others.

In the last few years, the internet has become an increasingly effective tool for uncovering the white identities of pretendians. It can be a little unnerving to watch story after story unfold in multiple public institutions of people who have gained access to positions of power and privilege based on what sometimes turn out to be overstatements of their Indigenous ancestry and other times turn out to be complete fabrications (Jago, 2021). It feels like the epitome of the word *scandalous*, complete with shame, recriminations, and all those comments in the *Globe and Mail*. I have been so set on edge by this at times that I have even found myself pulling out the family genealogy I used when I applied for my membership with Métis Nation of British Columbia (MNBC), just to reassure myself that I am not making up my identity, that the locus of my professional drive is rooted in a firm reality. I am, indeed, as my uncle has asserted, Métis—Métis enough.

But my concerns are not so unusual in the broader context of navigating Indigenous identities in Canada. Vowel (2016) has expressed her frustration and eventual exhaustion with repeatedly having not only to explain her own identity as a Métis Iskwew but also the notion of this identity writ large within the colonial history of Turtle Island. As Adese et al. (2017) assert, "in many ways, the Métis are at the frontlines of navigating the complex terrain of Indigeneity in Canada, with Métis identity consistently, and often uncritically mediated through the courts, through public opinion, and the media, rather than through Métis communities and peoples themselves" (p. 4). It can feel, sometimes, like we are constantly under suspicion and on the defensive, performing at an adjudicated dance recital that never ends.

It is easy to fall too deeply into these dark aspects of navigating Indigenous identities; to let imposter syndrome, lateral violence, and microaggressions taint my relationship to myself and to the work I am called to do. As Bhattacharya (2016) points out, "well-intentioned colleagues may be unaware of their roles in creating and reinforcing dominant, imperialistic grand narratives" (p. 316). And while it is good to know that there is some acknowledgement of this reality in academia, that doesn't take away the sting when it happens or the scars and trigger points it leaves behind. It is easy to feel small in a large public institution that demands I be certain things at select times while simultaneously punishing me for being those things at other times or for not being enough of those things that are expected of me in general. It is tempting to daydream about giving it all up to write young adult fiction or sell shoes, because some days it feels like *anything* would be better for my soul than what I am actually doing. But those are the bad days, the bad colonial days when cognitive imperialism (Battiste & Henderson, 2009) wins out over the teachings in my blood and my heart and my mind. Those are the days when there isn't any music or any reason to dance at all. I maintain, however, that being Métis in the academy is actually a power position. In the next section, I demonstrate the ways in which this is so by discussing how we can be the embodiment of two-eyed seeing (Bartlett et al., 2012), of serving as an ontological bridge between Western and Indigenous worlds, of the importance of being an academic auntie, and of the power of speaking back.

Teaching from Two Worlds

One of the first things I teach in my required course in Indigenous education is the way in which many Canadians take up what Susan Dion (2007) calls "perfect stranger" positioning. That is, the curriculum that has been delivered in Canadian schools over the past century and a half has been deliberately designed to historicize, minimize, and even erase Indigenous histories and presence from textbooks and curricular materials and consequently from the Canadian psyche. It is the nurturing of this grand national ignorance that has allowed the colonial project to continue and even thrive as falsehoods, stereotypes, and colonial mythologies have taken the place of truth and genuine relations (Donald, 2009, 2019). I begin in this way to get at the reasons so many in- and pre-service teachers are anxious about and even resistant to including Indigenous content and resources in their classrooms—they don't know much because they weren't taught much (Dion, 2007; Schick & St. Denis, 2003). In fact, we were all deliberately miseducated so that the colonial mythologies and stereotypes that fuel the colonial project could keep finding room to grow. This is glaringly true in the discussion of Indigenous identity in general and Métis identity in particular. As Vowel (2016) notes, these mythologies and stereotypes have significantly muddied the waters with status, blood quantum, and enfranchisement. Worse, such discussions were never included in school curriculum, almost as if misinformation regarding Indigenous peoples and histories was the goal of education.

And yet, in many provinces, Indigenous content is now a required part of curriculum. So where are teachers supposed to begin to unlearn being a perfect stranger and relearn the truth? Who is going to help them? And what should that help look like? One of the biggest "Aha!" moments for my students often comes when I start to talk about the differences between Indigenous and Western ontologies. I use a triangle to point to the anthropocentric and hierarchical nature of non-Indigenous conceptions of the world and a circle to point to the holistic and relational conception of the world that are characteristic of most Indigenous peoples. In revealing this fundamental difference, teacher candidates, an overwhelming majority of whom are non-Indigenous and come largely from white and Asian families, begin to understand that our differences are more than skin deep but extend to the very land itself (Simpson, 2012). They begin to understand the colonial logic of resource extraction versus a stewardship of balance, of seeing the land as a site for recreation versus seeing the land as a teacher (Seawright, 2014), of notions of owning the land versus notions of belonging to the land, of kinship extending beyond genealogy to all of our more-than-human relations.

This can produce tremendous discomfort for those who have not begun to grapple with their own place in colonization. For many, it is a complex new dance to learn, and the going can be tough. Because the positivist thinking that has long influenced Western ontology (Michell, 2018) tends to be binary (right or wrong, yes or no, all or none), some teacher candidates experience cognitive dissonance and even feel threatened. They mistakenly assume they are being told that they are completely wrong and must give up all of their most closely held beliefs. They worry that they will be forced to replace their worldview with Indigenous thinking, which ironically always seems foreign to them. I don't say this with unkindness—my observations are based on my own research (Leddy & O'Neill, 2021) and the work of Schick and St. Denis (2005), Ladson-Billings (2003), and a host of others who have seen it play out time and time again. This binary thinking is part of what makes it easy for settler folks to say, "so you're only a little bit Métis, a little bit Indigenous." This summer, when visiting the Back to Batoche Festival in Saskatchewan for the first time, I was surrounded by my prairie relations. It is true, as Vowel (2016) points out, that we come in all shapes and sizes—and all of us were more than a little bit Métis.

Bringing Indigenous Pedagogies and Frameworks to the Dance Floor

This, I think, is where being Métis begins to come in very handy. Being born from two cultures means being the embodiment of what Miqmaq scholars Albert and Murdena Marshall (Bartlett et al., 2012) have called two-eyed-seeing; that is, it is the gift of being able to see the world with one eye through the lens of all the best that Western thinking has to offer while the other eye sees through the lens of all the best Indigenous thinking has to offer. Originally conceived as an approach to Indigenous science education at Memorial University, in the context of teacher education it means bringing the awareness that there are—at least—two equally legitimate ontologies at play in this country to bear in the classroom. Especially as a guest on Musqueam land, it also means making clear that my Saskatchewan Métis ways are different those of my coastal cousins; we are not a monolith.

In pedagogical terms, teaching the concept of two-eyed seeing means helping teacher candidates explore what implications this understanding might have in classroom practice. It means helping them find a pathway to the seven sacred teachings (love, truth, humility, honesty, wisdom, courage and respect) so they can make space within themselves to hold both visions. It means unpacking the notion of seven generations in relation to *all* of us so we can think through how we have come to be where we are and figure out where we need to go next—and to go there together. It means introducing Indigenous pedagogies such as storywork (Archibald, 2008), circle work (Graveline, 1998), experiential learning, and holistic frameworks across curricular areas and demonstrating how they have parallels with some Western approaches, most of which we just call "best practices." It means drawing from as many communities as possible, introducing the medicine wheel as a holistic framework that considers how lessons can meet students in all quadrants: intellectual, spiritual, emotional, and physical (Bopp et al., 1989) It means serving as a bridge.

Being an Academic Auntie

We come to understand our Indigenous ways through relationships. We learn from our parents, our tantes et des oncles, our Kokums and Mosoms, les cousins, and those who look like us and sound like us. We learn through taking part in the chores of daily life, by watching, by practicing. We learn through ceremony, through stories, through our dreaming. And those of us who pursue careers that require higher education also learn about our Western ways through study, reading, seminars and lectures, citation styles, and writing. We have the opportunity to learn how our two ways are similar and about how our two ways are different. We have the gift of seeing things through both eyes and the gift of imagining how we could be better using both together. And we have the responsibility to do the work to make that happen.

Being Métis in the academy means you have enough resilience to survive the micro-aggressions from professors, classmates, and staff whose "no offense" usually means that offense is precisely what is coming (Bhattacharya, 2016). It means becoming familiar with the phrases and moves to innocence that mean you are less important, less believable, and less deserving of any gains you may make. It means understanding the value of healing and kindness and seeking to build relationships with those who are on the same good path, and it means reaching out to those coming up and supporting them as they too learn these things—being an academic auntie or uncle of sorts.

Being that auntie or uncle also means working for change. It means noticing when our relations are struggling and making sure we have enough backbone to help them. It means learning when to wait and watch and listen and knowing when to speak the truth. We have to be prepared to get our elbows up and make space for ourselves at the table. As Cardinal-Schubert (2004) aptly puts it, "let making a noise be truly our OWN NOISE rather than a bad imitation of a bad imitation. Let it be a clear song of the lands we come from. We have always been here. Our artists have always been here" (p. 34).

Then we need to hold that space for those who will come after us. That means using two eyed-seeing to critique and dismantle colonial practices that regard our ontologies as incommensurable. Sometimes it might even mean working as an ambassador for both sides so we can find the third space (Bhabha & Rutherford, 2006) of ethical relationality (Donald, 2009). We have to remember to nourish and care for ourselves as we nourish and care for others—you can't feed a family from an empty pot. We need to uphold the ethic of "nothing about us without us"; Indigenous voices need to represent

Indigenous thinking and stories. It is too late in the day for anything else. And, of course, we need to love everybody up with food. I'll bring the bannock, you bring the jam and Cheez Whiz.

Keep on Dancing

Although I did not meet my father and his family until I was in my 30s, growing up in Saskatoon I found enough welcome and acceptance amongst Indigenous friends to learn what I needed to know without knowing exactly what community would claim me as Indigenous. Once I learned more about who I am and where I am from, I was able to fully devote myself to working to improve relations between Indigenous and non-Indigenous Canadians. Currently, my role involves teaching Indigenous education courses to pre-service teachers, and I work hard to make sure I am honoring all those who have been willing to teach me. I maintain strong cultural and social connections with my Indigenous colleagues at UBC. I also continue to learn from my dad's brothers and sisters, most of whom remain strongly connected to their Métis heritage and traditions. My uncle Dan Kane, the one from the story at the beginning, in particular has shared many of his teachings with me and continues to help me learn about our family, our history, and our culture. It is possible to dance in two worlds, and I will continue to do so in the service of lifting us all.

References

Adese, J., Todd, Z., & Stevenson, S. (2017). Mediating Métis identity: An interview with Jennifer Adese and Zoe Todd. *MediaTropes*, 7(1), 1–25. https://mediatropes.com/index.php/Mediatropes/article/view/29157/21708

Archibald, J. A. (2008). *Indigenous storywork: Educating the heart, body, mind, and spirit*. UBC Press.

Bartlett, C., Marshall, M., & Marshall, A. (2012). Two-eyed seeing and other lessons learned within a co-learning journey of bringing together Indigenous and mainstream knowledges and ways of knowing. *Journal of Environmental Studies and Sciences*, 2(4), 331–340. https://doi.org/10.1007/s13412-012-0086-8

Battiste, M., & Henderson, J. (S.) Y. (2009). Naturalizing Indigenous knowledge in Eurocentric education. *Canadian Journal of Native Education*, 32(1). https://doi.org/10.14288/cjne.v32i1.196482

Bhabha, H. K., & Rutherford, J. (2006). Le tiers-espace: Entretien avec Jonathan Rutherford [The third space: Interview with Jonathan Rutherford]. *Multitudes*, 26(3), 95–107. https://www.multitudes.net/Le-Tiers-espace-Entretien-avec/

Bhattacharya, K. (2016). The vulnerable academic: Personal narratives and strategic de/colonizing of academic structures. *Qualitative Inquiry*, 22(5), 309–321. https://doi.org/10.1177/1077800415615619

Bopp, M., Brown, L., Lane, P. (1989). *The sacred tree*. Four Worlds International Institute for Human and Community Development.

Cardinal-Schubert, J. (2004). Flying with Louis. In L. A. Martin (Ed.), *Making a Noise! Aboriginal Perspectives on Art, Art History, Critical Writing, and Community* (pp. 26–49). Walter Phillips Gallery.

Cyca, M. (2022, September 6). The curious case of Gina Adams: A "pretendian" investigation. *Maclean's*. https://macleans.ca/longforms/the-curious-case-of-gina-adams-a-pretendian-investigation/

Dion, S. (2007). Disrupting moulded images: Identities, responsibilities and relationships – Teachers and Indigenous subject material. *Teaching Education*, 18(4), 329–342. https://doi.org/10.1080/10476210701687625

Donald, D. (2009). Forts, curriculum, and Indigenous Métissage: Imagining decolonization of Aboriginal-Canadian relations in educational contexts. *First Nations Perspectives*, 2 (1), 1–24. https://mfnerc.org/wp-content/uploads/2022/10/004_Donald.pdf

Donald, D. (2019). Homo economicus and forgetful curriculum. In H. Tomlins-Jahnke, S. D. Styres, S. Lilley, & D. Zinga (Eds.), *Indigenous education: New directions in theory and practice* (pp. 103–125). University of Alberta Press.

Graveline, F. J. (1998). *Circle works: Transforming Eurocentric consciousness*. Fernwood.

Jago, R. (2021, February 1). Criminalizing "pretendians" is not the answer: We need to give First Nations control over grants. *National Post*. https://nationalpost.com/opinion/robert-jago-criminalizing-pretendians-is-not-the-answer-we-need-to-give-first-nations-control-over-grants

Ladson-Billings, G. (2003). It's your world, I'm just trying to explain it: Understanding our epistemological and methodological challenges. *Qualitative Inquiry*, 9(1), 5–12. https://doi.org/10.1177/1077800402239333

Leddy, S. & O'Neill, S. (2021). It's not just a matter of time: Exploring resistance to Indigenous education. *Alberta Journal of Educational Research*, 67(4), 336–350. https://doi.org/10.11575/ajer.v67i4.69086

Seawright, G. (2014). Settler traditions of Place: Making explicit the epistemological legacy of White supremacy and settler colonialism for place-based education. *Educational Studies*, 50(6), 554–572. https://doi.org/10.1080/00131946.2014.965938

Schick, C., & St. Denis, V. (2005). Troubling national discourses in anti-racist curricular planning. *Canadian Journal of Education/Revue canadienne de l'éducation*, 28(3), 295–317. https://doi.org/10.2307/4126472

Simpson, L. B. (2014). Land as pedagogy: Nishnaabeg intelligence and rebellious transformation. *Decolonization: Indigeneity, Education & Society*, 3(3). https://jps.library.utoronto.ca/index.php/des/article/view/22170

Vowel, C. (2016). *Indigenous writes: A guide to First Nations, Métis, and Inuit issues in Canada*. Portage & Main Press.

· 4 ·

THE MÉTIS NATION, EPISTEMIC INJUSTICE, AND SELF-INDIGENIZATION

Kurtis Boyer and Paul Simard Smith[1]

Introduction

There have been several discussions in recent years about the growing phenomenon of settler Canadians falsely identifying themselves as Indigenous (Andersen, 2014; Couturier, 2020; Donovan, 2018; Gaudry & Andersen, 2016; Gaudry & Leroux, 2017; Leroux, 2019; Pedri-Spade, 2022; Sturm, 2011). This phenomenon is often labeled "settler self-indigenization" or a form of "race-shifting" akin to the Rachel Dolezal case, in which a white woman claimed to be of African American descent. While self-indigenizers may come to associate their newly acquired Indigenous identity with any of the Indigenous peoples of North America, in the Canadian context specifically, when settlers shift to an Indigenous identity, they often claim to be some kind of "new Métis" (Leroux, 2019).

The goal of this paper is to propose a characterization of the concept of settler self-indigenization and to consider some of the injustices that are generated by settlers identifying as Métis in the process of self-indigenization. In particular, our aim here is to focus on injustices that come into view through employing an epistemic injustice lens. In the context of this paper, such a lens focuses on how deficient conceptual resources in the Canadian public's social understanding of the Métis are exploited by self-indigenizers as part of the rationalization of the process of self-indigenization. Achieving these goals, we believe, makes a contribution to a growing understanding of self-indigenization as a contemporary dimension of settler colonialism.

To begin, we provide a general background on the Métis nation, after which we offer a brief discussion of the concept of epistemic injustice. Next, we develop a conceptual analysis of the notion of self-indigenization. In the sections that follow, we outline the origination of various misconceptions and deficiencies in the Canadian public's understanding of who the Métis are and explain how these misconceptions amount to a form of epistemic injustice that renders self-indigenization more likely to occur and that undermines Métis self-government. By interrogating the epistemic environment that helps facilitate certain cases of self-indigenization, we hope to arrive at a clearer picture of some of the social mechanisms that underlie this contemporary dimension of settler colonialism and the injustices it generates.

Background and Core Concepts

Who Are the Métis?

We draw on our understanding of the Métis as a people, an understanding that is in line with one articulated by Chelsea Vowel (2016a, 2016b) and Chris Andersen (2014). A helpful statement that encapsulates the understanding we have in mind is that "the Métis are a post-contact Indigenous People with roots in the historic Red River community" (Vowel, 2016b). This people possesses internationally acknowledged markers of nationhood including; unique languages, foods, artistic styles, and a territorial homeland, distinctive kinship structures, legal and governance traditions, and most crucially political self-awareness as a distinctive people. The Métis have played and continue to play an important role in the history of the Northwestern Plains of North America. It is this distinctive people that we refer to when using the term "Métis."

What Is Epistemic Injustice?

We intend to bring into contact discussions of epistemic injustice, as it is found in the political theory and social epistemology literature, with discussions of settler self-indigenization. Thus, as part of setting the stage, we provide a brief overview of the relevant aspects of the concept of epistemic injustice.

To begin, it is worth reflecting on how it is possible for someone to be harmed with respect to different capacities. For example, they can be harmed in their capacity to earn a living, in their health or physical wellbeing, in their capacity to pursue their vision of what is good in life, or—and this is of significance to us here—in their capacities as a knower and interpreter of their own social experiences. Epistemic injustice pertains to this latter capacity in which someone can be harmed; it includes various kinds of unwarranted harms that occur to individuals and groups in their capacity as knowers.

Following Miranda Fricker (2007), there are two kinds of epistemic injustice that are in focus here. *Testimonial* epistemic injustice occurs when "prejudice causes someone to give a deflated level of credibility to a speaker's word" (Fricker, 2007, p. 1). In these cases, prejudicial stereotypes result in the assignment of a lower level of credibility to some testifier than is warranted. The other form of epistemic injustice that we consider here is *hermeneutical injustice*, which might also be called simply interpretive injustice. This results from widespread misunderstanding—what is known as conceptual or epistemic environment—among a dominant social group that undercuts a marginalized social group's capacity to interpret its own social reality and project this understanding onto the dominant group. More specifically, this kind of epistemic injustice occurs when there is a flawed epistemic or conceptual environment among a dominant group within a society. This environment operates so as to undercut a marginalized collective's capacity to enforce its own understanding of its social experiences.

What Is Self-Indigenization?

Further laying the foundations of our argument, we propose a characterization of settler self-indigenization, a phenomenon that has been characterized as a sudden decision to "identify as Indigenous without official recognition" (Couturier, 2020, para. 1). However, such characterizations are general, and there is room for a more precise formulation; thus, we propose a definition of self-indigenization for further consideration and discussion and try to provide some of the motivation for that definition.

> *Self-indigenization* is a process by which an individual comes to assert an Indigenous identity based solely on their view of themselves as Indigenous, without belonging to any Indigenous people.

There are several points that could be made about different aspects of this proposed definition, but here we consider *some* of the motivations for a definition of this nature. First, we begin by reflecting on the conditions in the world that if satisfied, would render a claim of belonging, or membership, to an Indigenous people true. To be clear, we are not intending to—nor do we—provide anything approaching a complete account of the truth-conditions for such claims. Instead, we simply draw attention to an essential feature that such truth-conditions must possess. In particular, the truth-conditions for such claims to belonging are *multilateral* in character. In saying that the truth-conditions of claims to belonging to an Indigenous people are multilateral, we mean that the self-understanding of the individual making that claim is not a sufficient condition for the claim to be true. The self-understanding of the individual making the claim must be reciprocated and reflected by the people to whom the individual claims to belong.[2] In general, the social facts that render claims to belonging to a collective true are not only determined by how individuals understand themselves but also about the collective's acceptance of that individual as a member. Regardless of the confused reasoning process or belief system that might lead someone to identify as a faculty member, a member of the RCMP, or a Canadian citizen, if they are not properly accepted by those collectives themselves, then their claim is simply false. The proposed definition of self-indigenization reflects that a true claim to belonging to an Indigenous people is, like claims to belonging to many other collective, multilateral in character; self-understanding or identification alone is insufficient.

Another important feature that motivates the proposed definition is that it distinguishes self-indigenization from cases where people know they are not Indigenous but say they are. Such cases, from a moral psychological perspective, involve lying on a serious matter and committing a kind of fraud. In cases of self-indigenization, someone may come to be self-deceived or to believe, in some sense, that they are Indigenous even though they are mistaken.

Having formed this distinction, it is important to clarify that because these two phenomena are distinct, that does not mean that one is morally speaking any less serious than the other. It also does not entail that the proper legal treatment of self-indigenization would not be akin to cases of fraud, for example, as Leah Ballantyne has recently suggested (Martens, 2021). What this does suggest is that at least from a moral psychological point of view, these are two different phenomena. Self-indigenization involves some confused and convoluted socio-cognitive process whereby individuals falsely come to imagine themselves as Indigenous, whereas saying one is Indigenous when one knows one is not is a flat-out misrepresentation.

The Epistemic Context of Self-Indigenization

There is a particular epistemic environment that has left the Métis at an epistemic disadvantage when enforcing the meaning and value of the word "Métis" on Canadian consciousness. The stories told about the Métis that have settled into the dominant Canadian public's social imagination contribute to an epistemic environment that leaves the Métis vulnerable to outsiders rejecting the notion of a distinct Métis nation, and it allows outsiders to define for themselves what it means to be Métis.

We home in on three stories about the Métis found in the dominant Canadian public's social imagination. These are the stories of treaty vs. scrip, of racial mixedness, and the liberal conception of freedom as non-interference. Taken together, these stories shape the Canadian public's social imagination of the Métis in a manner that undermines Métis individuals and Métis collective self-determination.

Relative to other Indigenous peoples, Canadians and the Government of Canada have consistently failed to hear the claims of distinction and nationhood that have risen from Métis communities over the years. The Métis assertion of nation-level distinction has consistently been met with a gap in understanding from the broader settler society. This gap originates, in part, from the narratives of racial ambiguity that have been directed toward Métis and through the ways they have been dispossessed of their land and thus deprived of the kinds of epistemic resources that are important for asserting a national distinction.

How Métis Are Excluded from Treaty Narratives

There are a variety of resources that a nation might have at its disposal when asserting its distinction to another group. Historically, signed treaties are one such resource. The idea that treaties are between two nations—a First Nation and the Government of Canada, for example—is an idea that lives on today through the popular phrase "we are all treaty people." In fact, the phrase and the treaty-making process have steadily become part of the political vernacular in Canada (McKenzie-Jones, 2019). Treaty-making is something that plays a role in creating a sense of self for Canadians. Treaties provide a common story and a sense of national birth. This serves as a powerful cognitive apparatus for maintaining a national distinction between Canadians and First Nations. For signatories, a treaty means that "identifying as a nation may be a non-issue. The nation has a continuing and profound historical presence and prominence in the minds of its people" (Cornell, 2015, p. 7). Treaties support external recognition of an Indigenous national identity and root a nation-to-nation relationship in the contemporary vernacular and cognitive landscape of society at large.

When the Manitoba Act was passed, there is very good reason to assume that at the time, many believed the Métis to be in a similar, if not identical, level of politico-legal authority as the Crown. Yet, even if the Manitoba Act came about through a peace negotiated between two political equals, the way the act came to be implemented in its purpose of "extinguishing Indian title" stripped the Métis of the kind of epistemic authority that treaties normally provide for asserting national distinction. In fact, the Canadian government carried out its efforts to extinguish Métis claims to land with the express intent of treating the Métis not as a nation but as individuals and wards of the Canadian state.

The extinguishing of title was carried out through a process decided by one party (the Canadian government), and the allotted 1.4 million acres of land were distributed at the behest of the Governor General to individual heads of families. In other words, the Métis dispossession of lands occurred through an individualization of land title. Compared to what treaties do for enforcing a nation-to-nation relationship in the Canadian psyche, individualizing the extinguishing of title is of itself an act that subsumes the cultural and national distinction of the Métis. Thus, the implementation of the Manitoba Act has meant that the Métis have not widely been acknowledged in the dominant society as participants in treaty agreements. For most Canadians today, the Métis are not considered "treaty people" in the same way that many First Nations are.

How Métis Nationhood Is Undermined by Racial Narratives

The "First" in "First Nation" makes an important distinction from other visible minorities in Canada. Unlike other minorities, First Nations have a historical claim to the land and their connection to it. In effect, and in a way that is similar to treaties, the very term "First Nation" serves to remind Canada that the history of its lands and peoples did not begin with European settlers and adds to the cognitive landscape that supports the idea of Indigenous nationhood for First Nations. Compare this with how the use of the term "Métis" has often become a conceptual placeholder for mixedness for many Canadians.

As noted, the Métis are distinct, "post-contact Indigenous peoples with roots in the historic Red River community" (Andersen, 2014, p. 27; Vowel, 2016). Like other Indigenous peoples, the Métis have their own languages, foods, art, dance, kinship networks, legal and governance traditions, and historical and political self-awareness as a collective distinct from European and First Nations. However, the Métis nation's ability to force a view of nationhood onto outsiders has been further diminished by the way that it has been subjected to a process of racialization.

Chris Andersen notes that the Métis nation has largely been seen by the Canadian public as a group made up not of a distinct culture, language, and social order but rather a bunch of racially mixed individuals, the offspring of two nations, one First Nation and the other European (Andersen, 2014, p. 6). This broader narrative of cultural ambivalence has made Métis nationhood vulnerable to being *misrecognized* as a hybrid offshoot of two races, "Indian" and "white," rather than as an *Indigenous* people full stop (Macdougall et al., 2012).

Compared to how the term "First Nations" clearly supports claims to nationhood, the fact that the word "Métis" acts as a conceptual placeholder for mixedness means that Métis nationhood must contend with a racialized hierarchy with political consequences. If First Nations are indigenous to this land, and if this provides them the moral standing for distinction and self-government, then because "only one half" of a Métis person come from First Nations, the Métis are only half Indigenous and, as a consequence, only half as deserving of self-government (Andersen, 2014, p. 7). Further, the idea that the Métis are a cultural offshoot more a kind of "first" nation unto themselves denies the Métis nation a powerful cognitive resource for asserting their distinction in the broader Canadian consciousness.

What and Who You Are Is Still Considered a "Personal Choice"

The notion that it is a "personal choice" or the individual right of a person to choose an identity is rooted deeply in the stories that liberal society tells us about human nature. Much of the liberal tradition, and perhaps political theory more generally, holds that people are born in a state of freedom. It is assumed that we are by nature free, making it necessary to justify any restrictions to that original state. There is no onus on individuals to justify their ability to be free to act in ways that represent their interests; rather, the burden is on those seeking to restrict freedom to establish justifiable grounds for doing so (Gaus, 1996, pp. 162–166). And the reason for this, it is ultimately assumed, is that our thoughts and actions are not predetermined but are transposed unto the world by an autonomous will—and self-awareness. Persons (2016), John Locke informs us, are in "a state of perfect freedom to order their actions (...) as they think fit (...) without asking leave, or depending on the will of any other man" (p. 287).

It is not uncommon for self-identified individuals and some settlers with decision-making authorities to invoke such conceptions of freedom and individual autonomy, which are often articulated in statements like "no one can tell me who I am other than myself," "I decide who I am," and "People have a right to identify however they like; who are you to tell them otherwise?"

Consequences

As a result of this epistemic environment, non-Métis are able to define what it is to be Métis in ways that suit their interests. This occurs on two levels: individual and group. As discussed below, each brings its own set of consequences for Métis people.

At the individual level, a growing number of identity fraud cases, particularly in the academy, have centered on individuals who have used their claim to a Métis identity to receive access to educational and professional opportunities. The rationalization of these claims commonly relies, at least in part, on invoking the stories found in the Canadian public's social imagination and detailed above.

On a group level, the inability of Métis to imprint the notion of their own distinctiveness onto the Canadian consciousness has allowed some non-Métis to define who the Métis are. For example, in his 2008 bestseller, *A Fair Country*, John Ralston Saul argues that contemporary Canada has been deeply influenced and shaped by Aboriginal and European ideas and experience for over 250 years. Indeed, it is the mixing of these two different experiences, Saul informs us, that Canada and all Canadians are part of what he refers to as a "métis civilization":

> We are a métis civilization. What we are today has been inspired as much by four centuries of life with the indigenous civilizations as by four centuries of immigration. Perhaps more. Today we are the outcome of that experience. As have Métis people, Canadians in general have been heavily influenced and shaped by the First Nations. (Saul, 2008, p. 3).

In discussing Saul's book, Andersen identifies the grand myth with which the very term "Métis" has been saddled:

> Despite Saul's scattering of references to various Métis national icons, swept up like so many autumn leaves into his larger narrative, the author's phrasing instead defines Canada's political history as hybrid and thus marks, perhaps, its—and his own—indigeneity. [Métis historian Brenda Macdougall explains that the problem] is that even presumably well-intended statements such as Saul's "instantly negate the stories of [Métis] families, the histories of our communities, and the authenticity of our aboriginality, reducing us to an in-between, incomplete, 'not-quite-people' who are stuck somewhere on the outside of the discourse." (Andersen, 2014, p. 5)

This is another example of the Métis being *misrecognized* as a hybrid offshoot of two races—"Indian" and "white"—rather than as an Indigenous people. More broadly, it is another example of the vulnerability Métis nationhood faces when non-Métis define what it is to be Métis. Saul's construction of Canada as a métis civilization is an argument made possible only because *he is free* to also ignore or downplay the ethnogenesis of the Métis as a distinct nation. Saul's assertion that Métis are "mixed" or "hybrid" is not new; nor is the process of appropriation.

The process of non-Métis people defining for themselves what it is to be Métis to advance their own arguments has led directly to obstacles to Métis self-governance. For example, Tom Flanagan adopts a highly dismissive position: "Métis self-government in any large-scale, meaningful sense is a nonstarter. Self-government requires territorial concentration of the sort that allows First Nations governments to exist on Indian reserves. But the Métis live all over Canada and are not likely to leave Edmonton, Saskatoon, or Winnipeg to set up remote self-governing enclaves" (2017).[3]

The argument that Métis self-government is impossible due to some kind of "demographic reality" is made possible only by Flanagan being able to first define the Métis in a way that suits his argument:

> The biggest of all problems is demography. The Métis National Council and its provincial affiliates claim to represent the descendants of the historic Métis of the fur trade. These were mixed-race people who worked for the Hudson's Bay Company

in what is now northern Ontario, the three Prairie Provinces, and the Northwest Territories. They have many descendants today, but they have also continued to intermarry with other races and ethnic groups. Marriages since fur trade days have given rise to new generations of partly indigenous ancestry. Striking a deal limited to the descendants of the fur trade Métis will prove to be impossible. The self-identified Métis are one of the fastest growing groups in Canada, according to the census. They increased from 179,000 in 1996 to 418,000 in 2011. The explosive growth is due to what demographers call "ethnic mobility," i.e., people changing the labels they give themselves. And behind the Métis are more than 200,000 self-identified non-status Indians who could plausibly claim to be Métis if they saw some financial incentive in it. There is, in other words, a pool of hundreds of thousands of people who may be drawn to seek official Métis status if these negotiations create a financial payoff to do so. "Build it, and they will come," as the saying goes. (Flanagan, 2017, para. 4–5)

When Flanagan defines the Métis, he does so as a racial rather than a cultural group. His ability to define the Métis in a way he sees fit and advance his straw person argument (to the detriment of the Métis aspiration for political self-determination) is not dissimilar to the process Saul employs when he advances his creation story of the Canadian state: both are based on a personalized appropriation of the definition of Métis. This process is made possible because of the way that the Métis as an Indigenous nation are structurally prejudiced by a gap in the collective Canadian understanding. The Métis have begun to address this gap by building institutions that allow them to force a national distinction on outsiders.

Conclusion

Relative to other Indigenous peoples, Canadians and the Government of Canada have consistently failed to hear the claims of distinction and nationhood that have arisen from Métis communities. The Métis assertion of a national distinction has consistently been met with a gap in understanding from the broader settler society. This gap, fed by the flawed stories told about the Métis that have shaped the Canadian public's social imagination, functions to undermine the Métis people's epistemic authority.

Rather than reflecting Métis people's authority in the determination of the truth of claims to being Métis, the Canadian public's flawed social imagination of the Métis permits people to determine the meaning and value of claims to being Métis in whatever fashion suits their interest and in a manner that excludes the Métis people. At the individual level, this produces a situation that makes self-indigenization more likely to occur. At the group level, the gap allows non-Métis to define what it is to be Métis in ways that undercut the Métis nation's pursuit of self-determination.

Notes

1. Both authors contributed equally.
2. It is important to appreciate that the relationship between many Indigenous individuals and the people they are from has been severely and profoundly disrupted by colonial state policies and by widespread attitudes in colonial society. Some examples in the Canadian context include adopting Indigenous children into non-Indigenous families away from their Indigenous community, the residential school system, scrip policy, and systemic discrimination. The effects of these policies and attitudes emanating from many settler people has contributed to many Indigenous people being disconnected from their own people. For such cases, inclusive membership protocols would hold such disconnected individuals to be one of the people. Thus, under these circumstances, where there is clear documentation of the state's policies and of their direct impact on Indigenous people, there is good reason for—and the general practice is that—Indigenous peoples to regard such forcibly disconnected individuals as members of the people that they are from. As Gaudry and Andersen note, First Nations and Métis membership codes commonly "contain provisions to incorporate those who have been disconnected from their people by colonial policy" (2016, p. 28).
3. There are also significant unsupported presumptions in this statement about the necessity of a conception of self-determination that adheres to the Westphalian model of statehood. For alternatives to a Westphalian conception of self-determination, see Nichols (2020).

References

Andersen, C. (2014). *"Métis": Race, recognition, and the struggle for Indigenous peoplehood*. UBC Press.

Cornell, S. (2015). Processes of native nationhood: The Indigenous politics of self-government. *International Indigenous Policy Journal*, 6(4). https://ojs.lib.uwo.ca/index.php/iipj/article/view/74757.

Couturier, C. (2020, April 7). Researchers examine the growing phenomenon of 'self-indigenization.' *University Affairs*. https://www.universityaffairs.ca/news/news-article/researchers-examine-the-growing-phenomenon-of-self-indigenization/

Donovan, J. (2018, February 20). Rampant settler self-indigenization poses a threat to Indigenous peoples. *Muskrat Magazine*. http://muskratmagazine.com/rampant-settler-self-indigenization-poses-threat-indigenous-peoples/

Flanagan, T. (2017, September 12). Métis self-government in Canada is a non-starter: Op-ed. *The Globe and Mail*. https://www.fraserinstitute.org/article/metis-self-government-in-canada-is-a-non-starter

Fricker, M. (2007). *Epistemic injustice: The power and ethics of knowing*. Oxford University Press.

Gaudry, A., & Andersen, C. (2016). *Daniels v Canada*: Racialized legacies, settler self-indigenization and the denial of Indigenous peoplehood. *TOPIA: Canadian Journal of Cultural Studies, 3*(1), 19–30. https://doi.org/10.3138/topia.36.19

Gaudry, A., & Leroux, D. (2017). White settler revisionism and making Métis everywhere: The evocation of Métissage in Quebec and Nova Scotia. *Journal of Critical Ethnic Studies, 3*(1), 116–142. https://doi.org/10.5749/jcritethnstud.3.1.0116

Gaus, G. F. (1996). *Justificatory liberalism: An essay on epistemology and political theory.* Oxford University Press.

Leroux, D. (2019). *Distorted descent: White claims to Indigenous identity.* University of Manitoba Press.

Locke, J. (2016). *Second treatise of government and a letter concerning toleration.* Oxford University Press.

Macdougall, B., St-Onge, N., & Podruchny, C. (2012). *Contours of a people: Metis family, mobility, and history.* University of Oklahoma Press.

Martens, K. (2021, December 1). Time to charge those pretending to be Indigenous with fraud: Cree lawyer. *APTN.* https://www.aptnnews.ca/national-news/time-to-charge-those-pretending-to-be-indigenous-with-fraud-cree-lawyer/

McKenzie-Jones, P. (2019, August 29). What does 'We are all treaty people' mean, and who speaks for Indigenous students on campus? *The Conversation.* http://theconversation.com/what-does-we-are-all-treaty-people-mean-and-who-speaks-for-indigenous-students-on-campus-119060

Nichols, J. B. D. (2020). *A reconciliation without recollection? An investigation of the foundations of Aboriginal Law in Canada.* University of Toronto Press.

Pedri-Spade, C. (2022, January 26). We are facing a settler colonial crisis: Not an Indigenous identity crisis. *The Conversation.* https://theconversation.com/we-are-facing-a-settler-colonial-crisis-not-an-indigenous-identity-crisis-175136

Saul, J. R. (2008). *A fair country: Telling truths about Canada.* Penguin Canada.

Sturm, C. (2011). *Becoming Indian: The struggle over Cherokee identity in the twenty-first century.* School For Advanced Research Press.

Vowel, C. (2016a). *Indigenous writes: A guide to First Nations, Métis, and Inuit issues in Canada.* Illustrated ed. HighWater Press.

Vowel, C. (2016b, May 10). Who are the Métis? âpihtawikosisân: Law. Language. Culture. https://apihtawikosisan.com/2016/05/who-are-the-metis/

· 5 ·

RETURNING TO CEREMONY: A MÉTIS SPIRITUAL RESURGENCE

Chantal Fiola

On April Fools' Day in 2022, Pope Francis addressed 200 Indigenous people who had travelled from Canada to the Vatican hoping to receive an apology for the Catholic Church's role in the residential school system. Speaking in Italian, the pope said:

> For the deplorable conduct of those members of the Catholic Church, I ask for God's forgiveness and I want to say to you with all my heart: I am very sorry. And I join my brothers, the Canadian bishops, in asking your pardon.(...) At the same time, I think with gratitude of all those good and decent believers who, in the name of the faith, and with respect, love and kindness, have enriched your history with the Gospel. (CTV News, 2022a)

That July, the pope delivered a second apology, this time in Spanish, in Maskwacis First Nation, Alberta, the first speech during what he called his "penitential pilgrimage" to Canada. He acknowledged that "children suffered physical, verbal, psychological and spiritual abuse" in the "disastrous error" and begged forgiveness for "the evil committed by so many Christians" (CTV News, 2022c).

These long-awaited apologies were healing for some survivors; however, many criticized the pope for not delivering them in English despite his ability to do so, for expunging the epidemic of sexual abuse in the schools (and the church's ongoing protection of predatory priests), and for "focus[ing] on the actions of a few members of the church" (Canadian Press, 2022; Palmater, 2022). Apologizing for an allegedly few bad apples who committed atrocious crimes against children conceals the Catholic Church's culpability as a key architect in the century-long genocidal residential school system. To "apologize" and in the same breath commend the church for the "good" it has done to "enrich" Indigenous history minimizes that genocide and its intergenerational impacts (BBC News, 2022).

The president of the Manitoba Métis Federation (MMF), David Chartrand, has taken a similar approach. Upwards of fifty-five MMF representatives visited the Vatican after the first apology, and despite being physically abused for speaking Saulteaux in a Catholic day school and wanting perpetrators to be held accountable, Chartrand asked the pope to "revive the churches" in Métis communities (Baxter, 2022; Monkman, 2021). He acknowledged unmarked graves in cemeteries at residential schools and announced an MMF investigation into Father Arthur Masse, a retired Catholic priest charged with sexually assaulting a female child at Fort Alexander Residential School in the 1960s, noting that he spent 20 years at churches in the Métis communities of Duck Bay and Camperville, Manitoba (CBC News, 2022). Two weeks later, the MMF shared photos of an archbishop surrounded by 25 Métis children in red robes after their confirmation at the church in Duck Bay.[1] At the 2022 MMF Annual General Assembly, a video was screened of Métis leadership praising the pope for his apology and letting them touch his hand but remaining silent on the devastating impacts of the schools and the Catholic Church's participation in them. Chartrand highlighted the Catholic pilgrimage to the St. Malo shrine in Manitoba and that the MMF replaced the cross with one made from wood they harvested in Jordan (D. Chartrand, 2022). Rushing past damning truths (without giving people time to grieve or heal) and pressuring Métis into reconciling with and recommitting to the Catholic Church risks retraumatizing people, especially since many Métis are not interested in church; one need only scan the comments on MMF social media posts for evidence.

These events have perpetuated the stereotype that all Métis are Catholic and do not participate in Indigenous ceremonies. In late 2021, when the Indigenous delegation to the Vatican was announced, the Métis National Council acknowledged that the Catholic Church had taken away Métis spirituality, "robbing us of sweat lodges and drums"; Chartrand challenged this statement, claiming these traditions had never been part of Red River Métis spirituality and encouraging Métis to recommit to Catholicism (D. Chartrand, 2021). Having researched Métis spirituality for 15 years, I knew Chartrand was mistaken and wrote a column in the *Winnipeg Free Press* refuting his claim, hoping to mitigate the damage it had caused (Fiola, 2022).

Below, I provide evidence—archival, oral history, and from the literature—that some Red River Métis people historically participated in ceremonies like sweat lodges, Sundance, and Midewiwin. I outline the Métis methodology I shaped to undertake interviews across two research studies, in which I spoke with a total of 50 Métis people who participate in ceremonies, and share selected findings. What emerges is a fulsome understanding of Métis spirituality, historically and in the present. We begin by locating the colonial roots of the stereotype noted above and consider how Métis people became intergenerationally disconnected from ceremonies.

History: Taking Aim at Indigenous Lifeways

With perceived cultural superiority, colonizers targeted Indigenous lifeways for eradication. Their efforts were mobilized through Christianity, day and residential schools, the child welfare system, and legislation like the Indian Act. These efforts (and their consequences) continue today.

In what would become Manitoba, itinerant and mobile missions began with the arrival of Catholic clergy in 1818 and continued into the 1870s (Fiola, 2015; Huel, 1996; McCarthy, 1990). When a location had enough inhabitants living there year-round, a sedentary mission developed into a parish (Fiola, 2021). Occasionally, Métis people would request a priest in their community. However, freedom of religion became compromised as Indigenous people endured increasingly overwhelming pressures to convert to Christianity.

While churches were responsible for the daily operations of residential "schools," they were funded by the federal government and aimed to "civilize," Christianize, and assimilate Indigenous people (P. Chartrand et al., 2006). Most Métis attended day schools, but some attended residential schools (Fiola, 2015). Day schools were run by the same clergy as residential schools, had the same assimilative agenda, and displayed similar patterns of abuse and intergenerational impacts (P. Chartrand et al., 2006; Fiola, 2015). A shift toward public schools occurred from the 1950s to the 1970s, as did the transition that led to the Sixties Scoop. Children with Indian status went from being stolen from their families and communities and placed in boarding schools to being placed in white, Christian homes. Non-status and Métis children, considered non-Indigenous by the government at the time, had been subjected to child welfare apprehensions for decades longer (Barkwell et al., 1989). The theft of Indigenous children continues: in Manitoba, 90% of children in care are Indigenous—the highest rate in Canada (Legislative Review Committee, 2018).

The 1876 Indian Act also negatively impacted Indigenous relationships with spirituality. One early amendment excluded "halfbreeds" from Indian status because the government denied Métis Indigeneity in their promotion of assimilation (Green, 1997). As punishment for the Northwest Resistance in 1885, Indian Act amendments banned ceremonies like potlatch, giveaways, and elements of Sundance and mandated fines, imprisonment, and the destruction of sacred items and lodges (Pettipas, 1994). When a 1951 amendment reversed the ban on ceremonies, Indigenous people were not informed and thus feared persecution for decades to come.

Ongoing colonial legislation of Indigenous identity and government-created divisions have become internalized by Indigenous people. According to the Indian Act (i.e., the federal government), band councils, and Métis governments alike, one cannot have both Indian status and Métis citizenship. The national definition of Métis adopted by the Métis National Council in 2002 requires that Métis be "distinct from other Aboriginal peoples" (2022). Children who have one parent with status and one with Métis citizenship are told they cannot be both. After generations of internalization, Métis and First Nations on the Plains have learned to ignore our considerable cultural, linguistic, and spiritual commonalities (especially among Métis, Anishinaabe, and Nêhiyaw; Fiola, 2021; Innes, 2021).

The consequences of colonial pressures to assimilate are widespread and intergenerational. The theft of our children has mirrored the theft of our lands through broken treaty promises and the failure to safeguard the 1.4 million acres of land promised to Métis in the Manitoba Act (1870). We have been forcibly dispossessed from our lands, cultures, and spiritualities, and many have forgotten their own relationships with ceremony. This is the origin of the pervasive stereotypes that Métis are Catholic and do not engage in ceremony. Thankfully, it is not difficult to find proof that our Métis ancestors participated in ceremonies.

Oral History, Written Records, and Contemporary Literature

Evidence that Métis people historically participated in ceremonies can be found in oral history, archival records, and contemporary literature. Métis Elder Maria Campbell confirmed this when I visited her in summer 2018 on her land near Batoche, Saskatchewan. Maria shared that she has been conducting ceremonies like sweat lodges and fasting camps for 20 years and that some Métis have been participating in these ways for as long as Métis have existed (Fiola, 2021). She introduced me to biographies about Gabriel Dumont, Riel's contemporary and the respected leader of the "Saskatchewan" Métis. Thompson's *Red Sun: Gabriel Dumont, The Folk Hero* (2017) details Dumont's extensive relationship with ceremonies: he was a pipe carrier and sweat lodge conductor who worked with medicines, smudged Riel's grave and mourners, and frequented Sundances (Fiola, 2021; Thompson, 2017).

At the archives of both St. Boniface and the Province of Manitoba, I combed through correspondence by the earliest priests to arrive in "Manitoba" and read their frustration regarding Métis who continued to participate in ceremonies whenever the opportunity arose. Writing in 1868, Father Charles Camper was discouraged to witness a Midewiwin ceremony in Duck Bay, a community of Anishinaabe, Métis, and some Nêhiyaw inhabitants: "They beat their drums day and night. The evening before they departed, a grand lodge was dressed. The complex ceremony unfolded. Every savage had their face pained with ochre."[2] The persistence of Indigenous ceremonies among the Métis can also be found in an 1866 letter written by Father Laurent Simonet, who was travelling to Duck Bay and encountered a well-respected Métis spiritual leader on his deathbed. Simonet wrote that the "sick person was an old Métis [Elder] but one who had lived his life as a veritable savage, believing and practicing all the superstitions of savages. He has always been recognized as a powerful ceremony maker."[3] Simonet applauded himself for converting the Métis Elder during the most vulnerable moments of his life.

Beyond oral history and archival documentation, a growing body of research illustrates the continuity of Métis participation in ceremonies. The MMF's own Pemmican Publications released *Metis Legacy II* in 2006, with Chapter 17 dedicated to Métis spirituality. Authors Darren Préfontaine, Lawrence Barkwell, and Anne Carrière-Acco criticize a sole focus on Métis Catholicism while ignoring Métis people's "traditional religion" (2006, p. 186). They discuss Métis birth and death ceremonies, feasting, spirit dishes, and Métis participation in Sundance through the Nêhiyaw-Pwat (Iron Confederacy), an alliance of Métis, Nêhiyaw, Anishinaabe, and Nakota in the early 1800s (Fiola, 2021). In another example, Métis scholars Anna Flaminio, Janice Cindy Gaudet, and Leah Dorion (2020) discuss contemporary Métis women's participation in full moon ceremonies and cultural teachings regarding fire bags, sewing, bison, and tea. I have also contributed to the dialogue on Métis reconnection with ceremonies.

Methodology: Centering Métis Identity, Communities, and Knowledge

In my first book (2015), I crafted a Métis Anishinaabe methodology that evolved into a Métis-specific methodology in my second book (2021). In the latter, I centered Métis sovereignty by ensuring that participants met the national definition of Métis, focusing on six historic Métis communities,[4] adhering to the MMF's Manitoba Métis Community Research Ethics Protocol, and hiring six Métis community researchers (Fiola, 2021). I began each study with prayer and ceremony (fasting and Sundance, respectively) and relied on medicines (tobacco and sage), including when approaching potential participants. I have spoken with 50 Red River Métis who have found their way back to the spiritual lodges of their (Métis) ancestors and participate in ceremonies today.

Shared Experiences Across Métis Communities

Below, I highlight selected findings, with a particular focus on *Returning to Ceremony*. Specifically, I touch on intergenerational Métis family relationships with Métis communities, religion, and spirituality, participants' personal spiritual journeys, and community-specific patterns.

Concerning Métis family relationships with Métis communities, multiple generations have lived in at least one of the six communities featured in *Returning to Ceremony*. Métis families are also connected to several Métis communities beyond those in the study (2021). One reason for this was the historic dispossession of Métis from our communities (like Rooster Town and Ste. Madeleine); when forced by colonial governments to move, Métis often relocated to another Métis community where they maintained kinship relations (Peters et al., 2018).

Regarding Métis family relationships with religion and spirituality, all but one person indicated a strong Catholic influence; however, a few also spoke of Indigenous spirituality while growing up. For some Métis families, adherence to Catholicism reflected a survival mechanism, as in this participant's story:

> The way to rise above the poverty, to rise above the discrimination, is to show how devout you were as Catholics. That was your *Métishood*; that was who you were. It had to do with being a choirboy. It had to do with being altar boys from a young age. It had to be showing up for church and having twelve people [from your family] fill up two pews, and then you were proud.(...) If you weren't Catholic, you would not, could not elevate yourself. You could not find work; there was going to be no hope out of your poverty and misery. (Fiola, 2021, p. 147)

Others were aware of traditional Indigenous spirituality in their family or Métis community while growing up. One participant noted, "I got a really big book (...) [that] goes into [great] length about Camperville and practicing the Midewiwin ceremonies and Sundance ceremonies [historically]" (Fiola, 2021, p. 148). Similarly, someone from Duck Bay shared the following:

> There were ceremonies held in my community. The shake tent was brought there by the elders. There's a certain part there (...) across the lake, they used to hold ceremonies there. In the 1800s, all the tribes from all around [went] there.(...) They brought shake tents there twice because two twin brothers drowned and they wanted elders to help them, wise men to find where the bodies went down, where they'd be.(...) [That] was in the 1950s. (Fiola, 2021, p. 148)

More than half the people I spoke with noted a decrease in or complete end to their family's participation in church and increased relationships with ceremonies (Fiola, 2021). Some Métis families have continued to honor Indigenous spirituality into the present.

Participants also reflected on their personal spiritual journeys, including factors that inhibited and/or encouraged a reconnection to Indigenous spirituality. The most common disconnection factors included the church or Catholicism, day and residential schools, and fear, anxiety, and self-doubt (e.g., not appearing "Indigenous enough" and internalizing the stereotype that Métis do not participate in ceremonies; Fiola, 2021). The most frequently reported connection factors included impactful people (friends, family, Elders, one's spiritual community), significant catalysts (illness, death, abuse), and, ironically, higher education. While day and residential schools contributed to the intergenerational separation of Métis families from Indigenous spirituality, higher education can now facilitate access to Elders, cultural activities, and ceremonies (Fiola, 2021). The Métis people we spoke with participate in many ceremonies (between two to sixteen types), especially sweat lodge, Sundance, smudging, using traditional medicines, pipe, spirit name, and fasting (Fiola, 2021).

Community-specific patterns also surfaced in *Returning to Ceremony*. Duck Bay, Camperville, and St. Laurent still have larger Indigenous than non-Indigenous populations (Statistics Canada, 2018). In those places, we observed stronger intergenerational residence patterns; that is, families living in the same Métis community for generations (Fiola, 2021). St. François-Xavier, Lorette, and Ste. Anne now have larger non-Indigenous populations (Statistics Canada, 2018), and residents of those places reported experiencing greater pressures to assimilate. They shared more stories about their ancestors being forcibly removed from their Métis communities (higher rates of mobility), had less knowledge of historic family connection to ceremony, and expressed more self-doubt and internalized stereotypes regarding Métis identity and spirituality (Fiola, 2021).

The final themes I note are that many Métis people continue to leave their (Manitoba) Métis communities to participate in ceremonies; however, ceremonies are becoming increasingly accessible in some Métis communities. Some individuals travel as far as Alberta for ceremony; at some point, they connected with a spiritual community there and remain loyal to it. Others spoke of overcoming challenges to hold ceremonies in Métis communities, as in the story below, which took place in St. Paul, Alberta:[5]

> I had told everybody, I'm going to be putting up red [prayer] flags at the four corners, the directions, to come to our place. So, they all found the place easily.(...) There was about 300 people that showed up. [After the fast ended,] I went to take down the flags to burn them [in a sacred fire]. And here they were all gone. So, I thought because I had put them at road signs that the municipality picked them up. So, I went to the municipality and said, "Did you guys pick up four red flags at four different intersections?" He says, "Yeah. One of your neighbours came to us and told us there was going to be an Indian uprising, all these Native people heading to your place." And I burst out laughing! I says, "Oh my god, next time you talk to him, tell him to come over for tea and ask [me about it].(...) If he would have had tea and bannock with us, we would have helped him understand what this was about. (...) People fear things because they don't understand [them]." (Fiola, 2021, p. 221)

While that story took place in a historic Métis community in Alberta, other participants travel to access ceremonies in non-Métis communities, including First Nation reserves.

We also heard stories of ceremonies becoming available (or returning) to Métis communities, including participants conducting sweat lodges, hosting culture or fasting camps and in one case Sundance on their property. A few years ago, Sundance *returned* to the community of Duck Bay, which is ironically David Chartrand's home community. In another example, a participant from St. Laurent shared a story about the local Catholic priest visiting while she was constructing a sweat lodge:

> When we built the sweat lodge [in my yard], the priest came. Father Michel was Métis; he would talk to me about spirituality and ceremony. He'd have sage in the house where he lived. I went and cleaned the sage for him one time, and I did some teachings about sage. He always said he wanted to know more, and he wanted to participate in ceremony. So, on the day that we were building the lodge, I had invited him. He came and dropped by with his holy water, and he [splashed] his holy water on the sweat lodge, on the ground. (Fiola, 2021, p. 188)

She clarified that Father Michel blessed the sweat lodge and was supportive of her conducting sweats in the community; consequently, other (Catholic) Métis residents participated in sweat, having heard that the priest gave his blessing.[6]

The Collective Work Ahead

Having had the privilege of listening to 50 Métis people who participate in ceremonies today and having confirmed (through archives, oral history, and the research literature) that Métis people participated in ceremonies historically, I conclude that it is time—actually, well past time—to end the harmful stereotype that Métis people do not participate in ceremonies. Métis spirituality exists on a continuum with Christianity (especially Catholicism) on one end, traditional Indigenous spirituality on the other, and syncretic blends in between. Métis spirituality includes ceremonies in its own right.

As I wrote this conclusion, there was much talk about the pending papal visit to the historic Métis community of Lac Ste. Anne (*Manitou Sahkahigan*, Spirit Lake), Alberta. Notices were sent out by the county to surrounding villages and towns, warning that Pope Francis's visit was expected to draw between 250,000 and 500,000 visitors to the small community—by comparison, their annual pilgrimage averages 40,000 people.[7] Well-known Métis artist and activist Christi Belcourt publicly criticized the organizers of the papal visit for failing to involve Lac Ste. Anne residents, paving a road just for the pope, and failing to erect a fence to protect Métis relatives in unmarked graves in the community.[8] As a result of this and efforts by local residents and Métis Nation of Alberta Region 4, some issues were addressed. The Lac Ste. Anne Métis Community released the following statement: "We are now in discussions with the church regarding infrastructure improvements at the pilgrimage site, protection of any unmarked graves, and involvement in the actual papal visit itself" (CTV News, 2022b). Belcourt responded with relief but noted several outstanding issues, including that "the church is the biggest individual corporate land owner in Lac Ste. Anne Métis community and it's currently selling off land to non native people." On the same thread, someone suggested that "an appropriate gesture of reconciliation, would be for the church to donate this land back to the native community," to which Belcourt replied, "[I] completely agree. Also, to stop hiding pedophiles in the church and insist they be prosecuted. And repeal the Doctrine of Discovery. This was minor and the big things remain untouched and unaddressed" (Facebook, July 15, 2022).

Many Métis are waiting for the pope to address these outstanding issues as evidence that the church is genuinely interested in reconciliation with Indigenous peoples. Likewise, the MMF has work to do, including holding the church accountable for past and ongoing wrongs against our people. As the national government of the Red River Métis, the MMF has a responsibility to listen to the concerns of all Métis, not just Catholic Métis. No one is served when Métis who participate in ceremonies are ostracized by our leadership, shamed, and accused of "identity shifting" (D. Chartrand, 2021). It is time that the MMF publicly acknowledge that for some Métis, ceremonies have always been part of *Métis spirituality*.

The pope has now come and gone, and his visit, the attendant media frenzy, and statements by Métis leadership have not deterred Métis from resolutely participating in ceremonies. This summer, many Métis worked toward their Sundance commitments, including my wife, who completed her third year. We've brought our daughter to both our Sundances since she was a few months old; now, she's nearly two-and-a-half and knows how to dance and when to raise her hands to the tree; she never passes up an opportunity to smudge when a helper brings one by. I am heartened to know our ancestors (who participated in these ceremonies) are smiling and dancing with us in the spirit world. My daughter, and every Métis person I've interviewed and ceremonied with over the past 15 years (many of whom are also raising their children in ceremony), give me immense hope. We are collectively healing the colonial and spiritual wounds of our people and remembering that ceremony can strengthen the Métis nation.

Notes

1. See MMF Facebook post dated July 3, 2022, and the June 6, 2022 edition of *Le Metis*, MMF's newsletter.
2. Centre du patrimoine, Lettre à Monseigneur Alexandre-Antonin Taché, de Père Charles Camper, Mission de St-Laurent, Lac Manitoba, 12 septembre 1868, *Les Cloches de St-Boniface*, vol. 25, avril 1936, 102–110.
3. Centre du patrimoine, Letter à Monseigneur Alexandre-Antonin Taché, de Père Laurent Simonet, St-Laurent, Lac Manitoba, 2 avril 1866, 7.
4. Duck Bay, Camperville, St. Laurent, St. Françoise-Xavier, Ste. Anne, and Lorette.
5. St. Paul, originally Saint-Paul-des-Métis, was founded in 1896 by Albert Lacombe as a Métis colony. A decade later, the community was opened to hundreds of white settlers, especially French Catholics. Métis still live there, but the dominant population is now of European descent (Statistics Canada, 2018).
6. I love this story about my mother's community that features a Métis Catholic priest who is encouraging of Métis ceremonies and a Métis Elder who conducts sweats on her property and ties the ribs of her sweat lodge with mini Métis sashes.
7. Comment by Chelsea Vowel on a Facebook post shared by Christi Belcourt (July 14, 2022).
8. Facebook post dated July 6, 2022, that generated 661 comments, was liked by 2,200 people, and shared 4,300 times.

References

Barkwell, L., Longclaws, L., & Chartrand, D. (1989). Status of Métis children within the child welfare system. *Canadian Journal of Native Studies*, 9(1), 33–53.

Barkwell, L., Préfontaine, D., & Carrière-Acco, A. Métis spirituality. (2006). In L. Barkwell, L. Dorion, & A. Hourie (Eds.), *Metis Legacy II: Michif culture, heritage and folkways* (pp. XXX–XXX). Gabriel Dumont Institute and Pemmican Publications.

Baxter, D. (2022, April 21). Manitoba Metis Federation meets pope, invite him to ancestral lands. https://winnipegsun.com/news/news-news/manitoba-metis-meet-with-pope-francis-at-the-vatican

BBC News. (2022, February 15). Dozens more graves found at former residential school sites. https://www.bbc.com/news/world-us-canada-60395242

Canadian Press. (2022, April 21). "He took ownership": Manitoba Metis meet with Pope Francis at the Vatican. https://winnipeg.citynews.ca/2022/04/21/manitoba-metis-meet-with-pope-francis-at-the-vatican/

CBC News. (2022, June 22). Manitoba Metis Federation will investigate priest charged with residential school sexual assault. https://www.cbc.ca/news/canada/manitoba/manitoba-metis-federation-father-arthur-masse-investigation-1.6497939

Chartrand, D. *President's message*. (2021, December 15). https://www.mmf.mb.ca/wcm-docs/news/lemetis_2021_12_15_20211222104914.pdf

Chartrand, D. *President's message*. (2022, September 1). https://www.mmf.mb.ca/presidents-message/presidents-message-september-01-2022

Chartrand, P., Logan, T., & Daniels, H. (Eds.). (2006). *Métis History and Experience and Residential Schools in Canada*. Aboriginal Healing Foundation.

CTV News. (2022a, April 1). Read the full text of the Pope's apology for Canada's residential schools. https://www.ctvnews.ca/canada/read-the-full-text-of-the-pope-s-apology-for-canada-s-residential-schools-1.5844874

CTV News. (2022b, July 14). Archdiocese assures Alberta Métis community that unmarked graves will be respected during papal visit. https://edmonton.ctvnews.ca/archdiocese-assures-alberta-m%C3%A9tis-community-that-unmarked-graves-will-be-respected-during-papal-visit-1.5988255?fbclid=IwAR2tZ1Qpa52z-bmokPc4USfWOlO-li4u7MGKlCwYklGzhZZtQlibiM5lF8w

CTV News. (2022c, July 25). Read the full text of Pope Francis' speech and apology. https://www.ctvnews.ca/canada/read-the-full-text-of-pope-francis-speech-and-apology-1.6001384

Fiola, C. (2015). *Rekindling the sacred fire: Métis ancestry and Anishinaabe spirituality*. University of Manitoba Press.

Fiola, C. (2021). *Returning to ceremony: Spirituality in Manitoba Métis communities*. University of Manitoba Press.

Fiola, C. (2022, January 3). Métis spirituality includes traditional ceremonies. *Winnipeg Free Press*, 3 January 2022. https://www.winnipegfreepress.com/arts-and-life/life/faith/metis-spirituality-includes-traditional-ceremonies-576001602.html

Flaminio, A., Gaudet, J. C., & Dorion, L. (2020). Métis women gathering: Visiting together and voicing wellness for ourselves. *AlterNative*, *16*(1), 55–63. https://doi.org/10.1177/1177180120903499

Green, J. (1999). *Exploring identity and citizenship: Aboriginal women, Bill C-31 and the "Sawridge Case"* [Doctoral dissertation, University of Alberta]. https://doi.org/10.7939/R3M61BW0P

Huel, R. (1996). *Proclaiming the gospel to the Indians and Métis*. University of Alberta Press.

Innes, Rob. (2021). Challenging a racist fiction: A closer look at Métis-First Nations relations. In J. Adese & C. Andersen (Eds.), *A people and a nation: New directions in contemporary Métis studies* (pp. 92–114). UBC Press.

Legislative Review Committee. (2018). *Transforming child welfare legislation in Manitoba: Opportunities to improve outcomes for children and youth*. Technical Report. https://www.gov.mb.ca/fs/child_welfare_reform/pubs/final_report.pdf

McCarthy, M. (1999). *To evangelize the nations: Roman Catholic missions in Manitoba, 1818–1870*. Manitoba Culture Heritage and Recreation Historic Resources.

Monkman, L. (2021, December 6). Manitoba Métis Federation president to ask Pope to revitalize churches in Métis communities. *CBC News*. https://www.cbc.ca/news/indigenous/mmf-metis-vatican-visit-pope-1.6275837

Métis National Council. (2022). *Métis nation citizenship*. https://www.metisnation.ca/about/citizenship (accessed March 11, 2024)

Palmater, P. (2022, July 24). Another pope's apology isn't enough when Catholic Church's cover-ups and hypocrisy continue to this day. *Toronto Star.* https://www.thestar.com/opinion/contributors/another-pope-s-apology-isn-t-enough-when-catholic-church-s-cover-ups-and-hypocrisy/article_54015d98-298d-554f-9c49-53a74331f7c0.html

Peters, E., Stock, M., & Werner, A. (2018). *Rooster Town: The history of an urban Métis community, 1901–1961.* University of Manitoba Press.

Pettipas, K. (1994). *Severing the ties that bind: Government repression of Indigenous ceremonies on the prairies.* University of Manitoba Press.

Statistics Canada. (2018, July 18). *Aboriginal population profile, 2016 Census.* https://www12.statcan.gc.ca/census-recensement/2016/dp-pd/abpopprof/index.cfm?Lang=E

Thompson, C. D. (2017). *Red sun: Gabriel Dumont, the folk hero.* Gabriel Dumont Institute Press.

· 6 ·

ARCHAEOLOGY WITH OUR ANCESTORS: THE EXPLORING MÉTIS IDENTITY THROUGH ARCHAEOLOGY (EMITA) PROJECT

Kisha Supernant, Emily Haines, Solène Mallet Gauthier, Maria Nelson, Eric Tebby, William T. D. Wadsworth and Dawn Wambold

Introduction

The history of the Métis in the lands known as Canada has often been told through the accounts of outsiders. Much of the scholarly literature has focused on how the Métis emerged from the fur trade as a mixed people, or a people in-between. While research over the last two decades by Métis scholars has exposed the racial and colonial underpinnings of previous historical accounts (Andersen, 2008, 2011a, 2011b, 2014; Devine, 2000; Macdougall, 2010), there remains much work to be done to tell history from a Métis perspective. Archaeological data have great potential to illuminate the daily lives of the peoples of the past, but most previous research on Métis archaeological sites has emphasized hybridity and creolization in material culture (Burley, 1989a, 1989b, 2000; Burley et al., 1991), rather than exploring these sites from a Métis perspective. Archaeology has much to contribute to the stories of the Métis past, as it can illuminate areas where the historical record is silent. The lack of previous Métis-led archaeological work inspired the creation of the Exploring Métis Identity Through Archaeology (EMITA) project, where elements of Métis ways of life are held in the belongings and sites of the ancestors; these are woven into the Métis kinscape, or webs of relations between families, ancestors, places, and other-than-human beings (Lakomäki, 2014; Macdougall, 2010, 2017). In this chapter, we share how different aspects of the EMITA project help articulate Métis rights and reveal deep historical connections to kinscapes in the homeland and demonstrate how the belongings of Métis ancestors can help tell our stories as Métis people.

From an Archaeology of the Métis to Métis Archaeology

While the lifeways of the Métis have been the focus of some historical research (Foster, 1978; Peterson & Brown, 1985; Sealey & Lussier, 1975), less archaeological study has been devoted to Métis-specific places, with a few exceptions (Burley, 1989a, 1989b; Elliott, 1971; Weinbender, 2003). The limited archaeology of Métis sites completed in the twentieth century tended to focus on the mixedness and hybridity of Métis material culture and architecture (Burley, 1989b, 2000) and was conducted without the involvement of the contemporary Métis community. The focus on "Métis-as-mixed" has been criticized by Métis scholars (Andersen, 2011b, 2014; Gaudry & Leroux, 2017), who argue that to reduce Métis to being "people in-between" undermines their personhood and nationhood.

In archaeological practice, the framework of Métis-as-mixed commingles with the settler colonial assumption and attendant narrative of Indigenous disappearance, assimilation, and elimination after European contact. The latter narrative has resulted in a severe underdevelopment in the archaeology of post-contact Indigenous presence globally (Byrne, 2003; Panich et al., 2018; Rubertone, 2000; Schneider & Panich, 2022), while for the Métis, it compounds the people-in-between narrative to cause widespread misrecognition of Métis material culture as belonging to Euro-Canadian or other Indigenous traditions (Farrell Racette et al., 2017; Hrycun, 2020). With this misrecognition of Métis places and material culture being so common, the Métis are often functionally erased from the landscape. In this way, archaeologists—intentionally or not—reinforce a version of history in which the Métis disappeared through assimilation into Euro-Canadian culture, clearing the land to be inherited by non-Indigenous settlers (Furniss, 1999). This version of history is not merely damaging and degrading; it is also patently false.

At the same time, archaeologists have been responding to Indigenous critiques of the discipline by increasingly conducting archaeology with and for

Indigenous communities (Atalay, 2006, 2012; Cipolla et al., 2019; Martinez, 2014; Nicholas & Andrews, 1997; Smith & Wobst, 2004; Supernant, 2018; Watkins, 2005), and more Indigenous archaeologists are conducting research on their own histories (Nicholas, 2010). The rise of Indigenous archaeologies has led to the development of theoretical and methodological approaches to archaeological research that are grounded in Indigenous ways of knowing and being.

One of the goals of EMITA is to shift from "archaeology of the Métis," an approach in which non-Métis scholars do work on our history, to a "Métis archaeology," where work is conducted "with, for, and by" the Métis (Nicholas & Andrews, 1997, p. 3). This is implemented in two ways. First, a major factor in this approach is the formal education of Métis as archaeologists. As members of the Métis community, we are best positioned to work with our ancestors, our communities, and our historic landscapes. Although this work is progressing, there are not yet enough Métis archaeologists to work on all the Métis sites to be found across our vast homelands. To address this while still conducting Métis archaeology, we have fostered meaningful relationships with non-Métis archaeologists, including several of the authors of this chapter, who are dedicated to working with and for the Métis. Listening to community needs, making research available to the community, and prioritizing the Métis point of view are all considerations that need to be embraced by Métis and non-Métis archaeologists alike for true Métis archaeology to take place.

Second, we are also questioning the interpretive frameworks of archeology itself. Archaeological research has typically focused on patterns within physical material culture left behind by past peoples, illuminating aspects of daily life and societies in the past through a variety of analyses that rely on categories of objects. Rather than concentrating on categories, a Métis approach to archaeology focuses on the relations between the belongings of the ancestors and their interconnections with human and other-than-human kin, including plants, animals, lands, waters, and spiritual beings. This interrelatedness is expressed through wâhkôhtowin, a nēhiyawēwin (Cree) concept, practice, and law (Wildcat, 2018) that Métis Elder Maria Campbell describes as representing relations of "human to human, human to plants, human to animals, to the water and especially to the earth. And in turn all of creation had responsibilities and reciprocal obligations to us" (2007, p. 5). An understanding of the Métis archaeological record through a Métis worldview necessitates centering the relations between the past, present, and future and between the lived experiences of ancestors and their belongings. We approach the belongings and places of the ancestors using a visiting methodology, or *keeoukaywin* (following Gaudet, 2019), by considering what it means to be a good relative to the belongings of the ancestors and to the living community. In the section below, we discuss how various elements of the Métis archaeological record can be explored using this framework, with examples from the Métis wintering, or *hivernant*, site of Chimney Coulee, located on the eastern edge of the Cypress Hills in southwestern Saskatchewan (figure. 1).

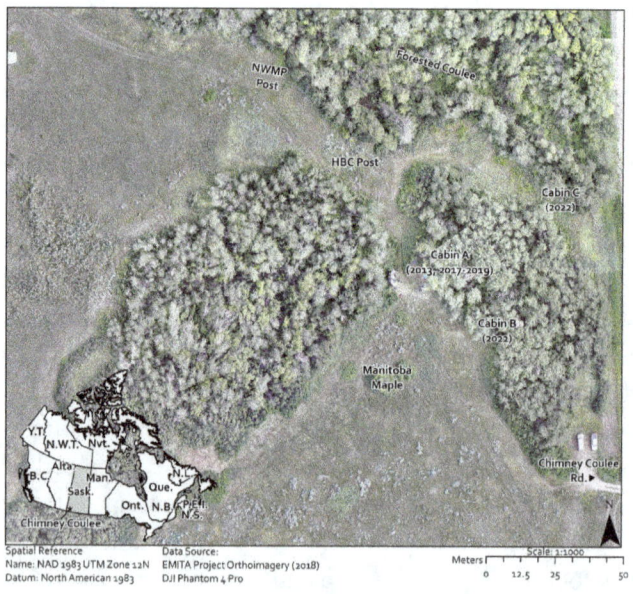

Figure 1: Site map for the Chimney Coulee Métis wintering site. Highlighted features are mentioned in the text; years denote excavation seasons.

The Ancestors of Chimney Coulee, Saskatchewan

Background

The Métis practice of hivernant developed over the course of the early nineteenth-century and expanded westward following the receding bison herds (D'Artigue, 1882; Macdougall & St-Onge, 2013; Sealey & Lussier, 1975). The tradition gained popularity across the entirety of the Métis homeland by around 1850 as the bison robe trade grew and provided additional economic opportunities for families participating in overwintering journeys. This gradual migration and expansion led large interconnected kin networks westward toward the Cypress Hills, along what is now the Alberta–Saskatchewan border (Macdougall & St-Onge, 2013). Oral histories suggest that the Métis were hunting and using the Cypress Hills as early as the 1860s and perhaps even earlier. Expanding from other settlements such as Wood Mountain and White River, multiple hivernant settlements along the hills began in the early 1870s, as the area provided adequate resources for hundreds of Métis families. The site of Chimney Coulee lies on the far eastern end of the hills near the modern town of Eastend, Saskatchewan. At its peak in the mid-1870s, the area around the Chimney Coulee site had approximately 400 Métis residents.[1] Most of the hivernant residents left in 1878 and relocated with their kin across the American border into northern Montana. A few Métis families remained at the site until the early 1880s, when it was permanently abandoned.

We began working at Chimney Coulee in the summer of 2013 with the intention of finding the precise locations of Métis wintering cabins. This involved testing a number of areas to look for historic material we could associate with Métis winterers and creating an updated map of the site. On the penultimate day of our field season, we came across materials—beads, ceramics, metal fragments, and so on—that suggested a Métis presence. We returned in 2017 to explore what indeed turned out to be a Métis cabin, opening an area that included evidence of a wall, with materials both outside and inside the cabin. Work continued on this building (Cabin A) in the summers of 2018 and 2019, where we used different techniques, including excavation, mapping, remote sensing, and near-surface geophysics to understand the cabin layout. While the work was on pause for two years due to COVID-19, we did return to the site in 2022 and used the same techniques to locate two other cabins.

Non-Invasive Methods

Our first goal when exploring the sites of our ancestors is to learn what we can without disturbing a site. Therefore, we begin by mapping out surface and subsurface using various technologies. The Métis structures and features that would have been built as part of the Chimney Coulee settlement are now mere traces and hard to observe archaeologically. The EMITA project has employed various non-invasive geophysical and remote sensing techniques to understand the subsurface and locate potential cabin features. These include ways to understand the site from the air and from the ground.

First, we used uncrewed aerial vehicles (UAVs, also known as drones) to fly over the entirety of the Chimney Coulee site using a variety of cameras and sensors. We took photos of the entire site to create an orthomap, where we can see the ground in high resolution through photography. This is useful for exploring areas without trees and producing accurate maps of the other activities we undertake. For areas with trees and bush, we use drone-based light detection and ranging (LiDAR), which returns a high-resolution topographic map of surface features and depressions that provides a detailed surface model for analysis and mapping. In 2019, we also used multispectral imagery, which highlights changes in the vegetation that may indicate areas of earlier activity. This was able to illustrate areas not easily visible on the surface, as activities in the past changed the social composition in ways that might not leave clear traces on the ground but do change the vegetation.

To date, several ground-based geophysical techniques to explore the subsurface have been used at the site to great success, including ground-penetrating radar (GPR) and magnetic gradiometry (Wadsworth et al., 2021). GPR, a geophysical tool frequently used in the large-scale mapping of buried walls and villages in ancient European towns (Trinks et al., 2018), was used at Chimney Coulee to locate the ephemeral wood cabin walls and associated materials like cabin clay and hearth features. Magnetic gradiometry, a geophysical technique used to assess the magnetic characters of subsurface objects, overlaid the GPR survey and was able to provide characterizing information, particularly concerning the clay from cabin walls, fireplaces inside the cabin, and metal objects like nails.

Other ground-based methods include high-precision global navigation satellite system mapping, in which we use satellite technology to obtain highly precise measurements on the surface. We use this to map the location of our grids for geophysical techniques and to identify where we want to begin digging. When we excavate, we also use total station mapping to be able to map where each belonging is located in the ground and any changes in the ground that help us understand the types of activities that took place there. These geophysical maps, while non-destructive by nature, allow archaeologists to better target where we want to dig, thereby limiting our impact (Mallet Gauthier & Wadsworth, n.d.; Wadsworth et al., 2021). Conducting targeted excavations based on these results allows us to explore the belongings of the ancestors.

Excavation Methods

Based on our initial findings in 2013, three 1 x 1 m square units at a confirmed Métis cabin were opened in 2017. The Métis occupation of the site is relatively shallow, so we tend to begin to encounter Métis belongings 5–10 cm below the surface and dig at 5 cm levels until we see a change in the soil. Belongings found in the ground are mapped in three dimensions; those too small to be easily seen are bagged along with the soil to be processed in the lab. In addition to excavation, we used geophysical surveys to delineate the cabin's walls and other features like fireplaces in 2018 and 2019 (Wadsworth et al., 2021). Small units uncovered wall and chimney features and verified the survey results, which led us to expand the survey to other areas of the site, where the remains of two fireplace chimneys and part of a cabin wall were unearthed during the 2022 field season. This has led to the uncovering of two additional probable Métis cabins: Cabin B and Cabin C.

Laboratory Methods

Excavations at Métis sites are distinctive in that the majority of artifacts cannot be retrieved using typical quarter-inch (6.35 mm) screen mesh. Previous researchers have highlighted this challenge but have also experimented with using window screen mesh that is small enough to retrieve the numerous <2 mm colored glass seed beads (Brandon, 2001; Doll et al., 1988; Weinbender, 2003). While time-consuming, this method of screening was used for every EMITA-led excavation at the Chimney Coulee site with considerable success. Over 3000 beads and hundreds of artifacts reflective of a domestic space have been recovered using this method and are vital to our understanding of Métis lifeways.

After belongings are uncovered, the next step is to take them to a laboratory for analysis. In a standard archaeology lab, this process can take on an air of impersonality in its quest for scientific objectivity. In the EMITA lab, we embrace the importance of scientific accuracy, but we also acknowledge that the artifacts were once the belongings of our ancestors. We recognize that these belongings have their own stories to tell. Our analytical methodology is therefore an act of visiting, or *keeoukaywin*, with the belongings to learn their stories. Through this process, we are able to discern the stories connected to these sites while acknowledging the emotional connections that we have with these landscapes and our ancestors.

Learning from the Ancestors: Interpretations

Métis Sense of Space: Site Layout

The multiple remote sensing surveys undertaken at Chimney Coulee have made clear that there are many more features still present at the site than originally thought. GPR and magnetic gradiometery surveys located at least two new Métis cabins, which were confirmed with archaeological excavation in the summer of 2022, and assisted with mapping the layout of Cabin A, which that was uncovered between 2013 and 2019. Many more potential structural features have been found in drone-based results. A new understanding of the site and its dynamics are beginning to form based on these surveys. Chimney Coulee was a large Métis site but was also somewhat cosmopolitan, with the presence of Northwest Mounted Police and Hudson's Bay Company posts (Brandon, 2001). Downhill from those posts were several Métis cabins clustered in a relatively small area. Each likely had its own features and may have been separated by family kinship groups, showing Métis relations. What is clear from our analysis is that there are many more areas to be investigated in order to understand the true significance of the site. Geophysics and remote sensing have allowed us to explore the site without overly disturbing the ground and has narrowed our focus in seeking to locate the belongings of the ancestors.

Métis Daily Life: Cabin A

One of the benefits of archaeology is that it can show aspects of people's daily lives. At Chimney Coulee, the lives of the ancestors are best captured through the belongings in and around Cabin A, the Métis cabin where much of our work has focused. Here, we were able to trace the wall of the cabin through patches of wood left in the ground. Outside the cabin, remnants of Métis life can be seen through many animal bones, primarily bison but also small mammals and fish from a lake that used to be nearby. Fragments of domestic items such as ceramics, glass, and metal have also been found. Inside the cabin, the pattern changes a bit, with fewer animal bones and more domestic items, including fragments of a number of different styles of ceramic cups and dishes that would have been acquired through trade. The belongings and the patterns they reveal clearly indicate that this was a Métis cabin.

In both areas, the most common belongings are small drawn-glass seed beads; overall, 3303 beads have been found to date in Cabin A. These beads

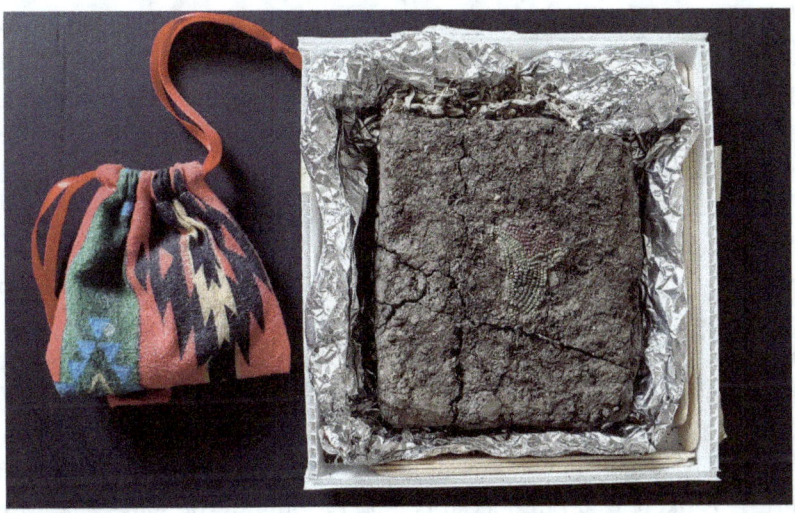

Figure 2: Métis beadwork found at Chimney Coulee site with medicines. Photo by Kisha Supernant.

are characteristic of Métis sites, but as noted above, we need to use specific methods to recover them. When we excavate with close attention to detail, we are also able to uncover some remarkable belongings. In 2017, team member Eric Tebby exposed a pattern of beadwork that was still intact (see Figure 2). This beautiful fragment of what was likely a larger garment shows a flower bud using colors and patterns typical of Métis beadwork. We were able to remove it from the ground and bring it back with us to the lab, where we care for it by keeping it with medicines and bringing it out to visit with relatives.

Métis Relations: Lives of Métis Women

Focusing our work on the cabins of Chimney Coulee has allowed us to explore the dimensions of domestic life at the site. The relationships and daily lives of women were of particular interest since they were routinely left out of the written records of the time. This exclusion was not necessarily intentional but was instead a reflection of the perspective of the primarily male authors and their intended audiences of other men (Van Kirk, 1980). The stories of our grandmothers, mothers, and aunties were revealed during our visits with the belongings that they left behind (Wambold, 2021). The tiniest beads, ceramic sherds, and fragments of personal items are telling us a great deal about our ancestors.

The kinds of women's stories the belongings are revealing can be found in the thousands of seed beads recovered from Cabin A. They tell stories of Métis women who were not only able to find the time and space to engage in beadwork but who were also able to build relationships with other members of their community. The detailed designs of the Métis women are not something that can easily be learned on one's own. It is a skill that is passed from one woman to another. For the Métis women of the past, it also required relationships with men to acquire the materials to create the beadwork. Through the many relationships involved in creating a piece of beadwork, we can see reflections of wâhkôhtowin and the reciprocal obligations within those relationships.

Many of today's beadworkers report that beading with others is an enjoyable way to pass the time and to build relationships with others in the community. It is likely that our ancestors used beading in the same way. Visiting with each other as they worked on their beading, the women would have been positioned to strengthen relationships within the hivernant community. Archaeologically, this may be seen as multiple discrete concentrations of discarded beads within the cabin walls, each concentration indicating where a woman may have sat to work on her projects. As was the case for bison hunting brigades (Hogue, 2015; Macdougall & St-Onge, 2013), female-centered kin networks governed the composition of overwintering settlements (Hogue, 2015). Women were at the center of hivernant contexts because of their key roles in the family unit and their role as connectors between different kinship networks. This is a key point, as those kinship networks have been described as being at the core of Métis identity (Macdougall et al., 2012).

Métis Connections to the Land: Foodways

Foodways are known across time and space to have played an important role in the definition of group identity (e.g., Hastorf, 2017; Twiss, 2019). This is also true for the Métis (e.g., Charette, 1976; Weekes, 1994). A few attempts have been made to relate the archaeological remains associated with Métis food practices to identity (Kooyman, 1981; McLeod, 1985), but mostly in ways that aimed to characterize Métis practices as different from those of other contemporary groups. The approach taken by the EMITA project allows for the exploration of the relation between Métis identity and foodways using newer archaeological concepts and methods, focused on understanding the social aspect of food and on Métis ways of knowing. The late-nineteenth-century overwintering Métis settlement at Chimney Coulee is a promising opportunity to explore what archaeology can not only tell us about what foods were eaten and how they were acquired and transformed but also provide a better understanding of the role played by food in the Métis world, particularly in the identity-building process and in its expression.

Societies express themselves through food traditions, such as recipes and the daily actions that meals create. For the late-nineteenth-century overwintering Métis, the relation between foodways and identity was also influenced by their environment. Indeed, while the overwintering Métis were active participants in the fur trade economy and sometimes relied on that trade to acquire staples like tea, sugar, and flour, much of their everyday menu was composed of wild foods, both animal and vegetal, that they acquired directly through hunting, trapping, and gathering. This relation with the environment was also a key element in the definition of Métis identity (MacDougall et al., 2012).

The importance of the role of women in overwintering Métis society, notably in establishing and maintaining kinship relationships, has been noted above but is especially obvious when examining descriptions of activities associated with food. While substantial attention has been placed on men and the bison hunts, much of the labor necessary for the survival of the family and the camp was women's work. These tasks included gathering fuel and food, hunting small fowl, and food preparation and cooking (Hogue, 2015). Through their plant-gathering activities, women also gained a particular connection to the land (Kermoal, 2016). This leads us to frame our approach to the study of foodways and identity in overwintering Métis contexts with a focus on women. Through their involvement in food production, preparation, and cooking, women expressed notions of kinship with the meals they produced. Therefore, we suggest overwintering Métis foodways can be seen as indicative of kinship relations and family traditions. Foodways also played a role in the definition of a broader Métis ethnic identity by unifying families and kinship networks around daily food acquisition, preparation, and consumption events, contributing to the perpetuation of traditions, the sharing of knowledge, and the creation and maintenance of social networks.

We are only beginning to explore what archaeological remains associated with food practices can tell us about the Métis hivernant occupation at Chimney Coulee. Nonetheless, tests and excavations at other wintering sites in the Métis homeland allow us to expect remains associated with the winter hunts, fishing, and trapping, dried plants (including herbs, fruits, roots, and spices), and possibly fresh plants and fruits collected at the beginning and

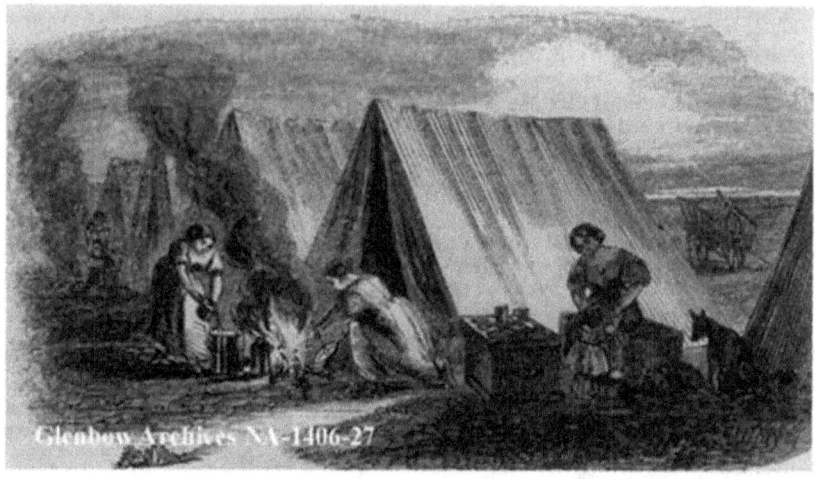

Figure 3: "Metis camp and woman baking, Pembina area, Manitoba," *Harpers New Monthly Magazine* 18, no. 104 (January 1859). Glenbow Archives NA 1406 27.

the end of the wintering season (Charette, 1976; Lyons, 2019). In the coming years, analyses of plant and animal remains, sediment samples, and other material culture elements (such as ceramics) will be undertaken so that we can learn more about the connection between food and the overwintering Métis identity during the late nineteenth century.

Moving Forward

Caring for the Belongings of the Ancestors

One important question for us is what happens to the belongings of the ancestors after we uncover them. Archaeologists in Alberta are required by law to eventually hand over all their archaeological materials to the Royal Alberta Museum, as archaeological evidence "within Alberta is vested in the Crown in right of Alberta" (Historic Resources Act, 2000), meaning that the government of Alberta is the authority on what should happen with any and all archaeological resources. The Royal Alberta Museum is the general repository for all archaeological materials within the province's borders. There, archaeological materials are labeled with identifying numbers called accession numbers, which allows future researchers to select specific things of interest. They are then stored in boxes and placed on shelves until someone decides that they are something of interest again.

For those of us who work with these artifacts as belongings in relation to our ancestors rather than objects, this does not sit well. As noted above, keeoukaywin invokes a promise that we engage with the belongings and by extension the ancestors to which they belonged. To learn their stories and send them away goes against the values that guide our research. Instead, we need to honor our own protocols and expectations about to remain in good relation with these belongings. This can include smudging them, placing medicine with them, and keeping them together. These approaches are often at odds with western academic frameworks and policies, as they do not consider artifacts to possess the same agency.

Furthermore, the process of surrendering these belongings to an institution like a museum only adds to the barriers that non-academic community members face. Community members have expressed the struggles of trying to gain access to our own material culture. Information about the landscape, what is above and beneath the soil, measurement, calculations, and the like face similar struggles of being locked behind gates. Often, the recordings of this information are unreadable to all but a select few and remain in folders on servers that may not see the light of day. What is to become of this information? Unfortunately, systemic change cannot be accomplished overnight, so solutions are required to help create bridges instead of barriers. One such way is the use of a database.

The creation of that kind of database allows for control over aspects such as data organization, accessibility, and information flow and dispersion. Involving the Métis community and giving them the ability to control the information enables us to engage with our belongings, even if virtually, and to situate them in our history and identity. It also allows for the integration of the spatial data to help form a more complete picture and understanding of these spaces and places on the landscape in relation to the belongings. We have our own ways of understanding and situating ourselves in relation to our past. Archaeological materials do not exist in isolation but contribute to the larger picture of connections between us, our past, and the land.

Métis Pasts for Métis Futures

The EMITA project is focused on reclaiming our stories. Métis history is beaded throughout the homeland, but far too much of it has been erased from our collective memory. We use the techniques provided by archaeology to help uncover what has been hidden and to reweave relations with Métis ancestors. By centering Métis ways of knowing in our work, we bring to life our past in ways that challenge how archaeologists have told our stories as Indigenous people. Ultimately, we do this work to build a brighter future for those generations to come after us, reclaiming Métis pasts for Métis futures.

Note

1 "Half Breeds are moving out from the foot of the Mountains for their seasons Hunt about four Hundred. Full riged out with Cayuses and red river Carts and Doges"–April 1877 (Clarke, 1886).

References

Andersen, C. (2008). From nation to population: The racialisation of "Métis" in the Canadian Census. *Nations and Nationalism*, *14*(2), 347–368. https://doi.org/10.1111/j.1469-8129.2008.00331.x

Andersen, C. (2011a). "I'm Métis, what's your excuse?" On the optics and the ethics of the misrecognition of Métis in Canada. *Aboriginal Policy Studies*. https://doi.org/10.5663/aps.v1i2.11686

Andersen, C. (2011b). Moya 'Tipimsook ("The people who aren't their own bosses"): Racialization and the misrecognition of "Métis" in Upper Great Lakes ethnohistory. *Ethnohistory*, *58*(1), 37–63. https://doi.org/10.1215/00141801-2010-063

Andersen, C. (2014). *Métis: Race, recognition, and the struggle for Indigenous peoplehood*. University of British Columbia Press.

Atalay, S. (2006). Indigenous archaeology as decolonizing practice. *American Indian Quarterly* *30*(3/4), 280–310. https://www.jstor.org/stable/4139016

Atalay, S. (2012). *Community-based archaeology research with, by, and for Indigenous and local communities*. University of California Press.

Brandon, J. (2001). The Regina Archaeological Society 2000 Field School at Chimney Coulee. Permit 2000-061. Saskatchewan Heritage Foundation.

Burley, D. V. (1989a). Flaked stone technology and the 1870s hivernant Métis: A question of context. *Canadian Journal of Archaeology/Journal Canadien d'Archéologie*, *13*, 151–163. https://www.jstor.org/stable/41102828

Burley, D. V. (1989b). Function, meaning and context: Ambiguities in ceramic use by the hivernant Metis of the Northwestern Plains. *Historical Archaeology 23*(1), 97–106. https://doi.org/10.1007/BF03374101

Burley, D. V. (2000). Creolization and late nineteenth century Métis vernacular log architecture on the South Saskatchewan River. *Historical Archaeology*, *34*(3), 27–35.

Burley, D. V., Horsfall, G. A., & Brandon, J. (1991). *Structural considerations of Métis ethnicity: An archaeological, architectural, and historical study*. University of South Dakota Press.

Byrne, D. (2003). The ethos of return: Erasure and reinstatement of Aboriginal visibility in the Australian historical landscape. *Historical Archaeology*, 37(1), 73–86. https://doi.org/10.1007/BF03376593

Campbell, M. (2007). We need to return to the principles of Wahkotowin. *An Archive*. https://mgouldhawke.wordpress.com/2019/11/05/we-need-to-return-to-the-principles-of-wahkotowin-maria-campbell-2007/

Charette, G. (1976). *Vanishing spaces: Memoirs of a Prairie Métis*. Editions Bois-Brûlés.

Cipolla, C. N., Quinn, J., & Levy, J. (2019). Theory in collaborative Indigenous archaeology: Insights From Mohegan. *American Antiquity*, 84(1), 127–142. https://doi.org/10.1017/aaq.2018.69

Clarke, S. J. (1886). *Clarke's handwritten diaries 1876–1886*. Glenbow Archives (M-229). Glenbow Museum.

D'Artigue, J. (1882). *Six years in the Canadian North West*. Mika Publishing. https://digitalcollections.ucalgary.ca/CS.aspx?VP3=DamView&VBID=2R3BXZQ1LE78E&PN=47&DocRID=2R3BF1FJN0CSZ&FR_=1&W=1920&H=919

Devine, H. (2000). Metis lives past and present. *BC Studies: The British Columbian Quarterly*, 128. https://ojs.library.ubc.ca/index.php/bcstudies/article/view/1549

Doll, M. F. V., Kidd, R. S., & Day, J. P. (1988). *The Buffalo Lake Metis site: A late nineteenth century settlement in the parkland of Central Alberta*. Alberta Culture and Multiculturalism: Historical Resources Division. https://www.electriccanadian.com/history/first/metis/buffalolakemtiss.pdf

Elliott, J. (1971). *Hivernant archaeology in the Cypress Hills* [Master's thesis, University of Calgary]. http://hdl.handle.net/1880/13577

Farrell Racette, S., Corbiere, S. A., & Migwans, C. (2017). Pieces left along the trail: Material culture histories and Indigenous studies. In C. Andersen & J. M. O'Brien, (Eds.), *Sources and methods in Indigenous studies* (pp. 223–229). Routledge.

Foster, J. E. (1978). The Métis: The people and the term. *Prairie Forum*, 3(1), 79–90. https://iportal.usask.ca/docs/Prairie%20Forum/The%20Metis%20(v3no1_1978_pg79-90.pdf

Furniss, E. (1999). *The burden of history: Colonialism and the frontier myth in a rural Canadian community*. University of British Columbia Press.

Gaudet, J. C. (2019). Keeoukaywin: The visiting way – Fostering an Indigenous research methodology. *Aboriginal Policy Studies* 7(2): 47–64. https://doi.org/10.5663/aps.v7i2.29336

Gaudry, A., & Leroux, D. (2017). White settler revisionism and making Métis everywhere: The evocation of Métissage in Quebec and Nova Scotia. *Critical Ethnic Studies*, 3(1), 19–30. https://doi.org/10.5749/jcritethnstud.3.1.0116

Hastorf, C. A. (2017). *The social archaeology of food: Thinking about eating from prehistory to the present*. Cambridge University Press.

Historic Resources Act. R.S.A. (2000). C H-9. https://canlii.ca/t/53q94

Hogue, M. (2015). *Métis and the medicine line: Creating a border and dividing a people*. University of North Carolina Press.

Hrycun, L. (2020). *Heart work: Weaving relationality into Métis material culture repatriation* [Master's thesis, University of Alberta]. https://era.library.ualberta.ca/items/f57f95a2-3115-4484-a56c-53f08b1e1034

Kermoal, N. (2016). Métis women's environmental knowledge and the recognition of Métis rights. In Kermoal, N., & Altamirano-Jiménez, I., *Living on the land: Indigenous women's understanding of place* (pp. 107–137). Athabasca University Press.

Kooyman, B. P. (1981). *Metis faunal remains and variables in archaeological butchering pattern analysis* [Master's thesis, University of Calgary].

Lakomäki, S. (2014). *Gathering together: The Shawnee people through diaspora and nationhood, 1600–1870.* Yale University Press.

Lyons, N. (2019). Palaeoethnobotanical analysis of Chimney Coulee (DjOe-6), Cypress Hills, Saskatchewan. Exploring Métis Identity Through Archaeology.

Macdougall, B. (2010). *One of the family: Metis culture in nineteenth-century northwestern Saskatchewan.* University of British Columbia Press.

Macdougall, B. (2017). *Wahkootowin as methodology: How archival records reveal a Métis kinscape.* Rupertsland Centre for Métis Research.

Macdougall, B., Podruchny, C., & St-Onge, N. J. M. (2012). Introduction: Cultural mobility and the contours of difference. In N. J. M. St-Onge, C. Podruchny, & B. Macdougall (Eds.), *Contours of a people: Metis family, mobility, and history* (pp. 3–21). University of Oklahoma Press. http://hdl.handle.net/10315/36814

Macdougall, B., & & St-Onge, N. J. M. (2013). Rooted in mobility: Metis buffalo-hunting brigades. *Manitoba History, 71*(13), 21–32. https://www.mhs.mb.ca/docs/mb_history/71/metisbrigades.shtml

Mallet Gauthier, S. (n.d.). Survey déjà vu: Lessons learned from the archaeological re-mapping of a Métis overwintering settlement. Submitted to *Canadian Journal of Archaeology*.

Martinez, D. R. (2014). Indigenous archaeologies. In C. Smith (Ed.), *Encyclopedia of global archaeology*. Springer. https://doi.org/10.1007/978-1-4419-0465-2_1

McLeod, K. D. (1985). *A study of Métis ethnicity in the Red River Settlement: Quantification and pattern recognition in Red River archaeology* [Master's thesis, University of Manitoba]. http://hdl.handle.net/1993/32303

Nicholas, G. P. (Ed.). (2010). *Being and becoming Indigenous archaeologists*. Routledge. https://www.routledge.com/Being-and-Becoming-Indigenous-Archaeologists/Nicholas/p/book/9781598744989.

Nicholas, G. P., & Andrews, T. D. (1997). Indigenous archaeology in the postmodern world. In G. P. Nicholas & T. D. Andrews (Eds.), *At a crossroads: Archaeology and First Peoples in Canada*. Simon Fraser University Press.

Panich, L. M., Schneider, T. D., & Byram, R. S. (2018). Finding mid-19th century Native settlements: Cartographic and archaeological evidence from Central California. *Journal of Field Archaeology, 43*(2), 152–165. https://doi.org/10.1080/00934690.2017.1416849

Peterson, J., & Brown, J. S. H. (Eds.). (1985). *The new peoples: Being and becoming Métis in North America*. University of Manitoba Press.

Rubertone, P. E. (2000). The historical archaeology of Native Americans. *Annual Review of Anthropology, 29.* 425–446. https://doi.org/10.1146/annurev.anthro.29.1.425

Schneider, T. D., & Panich, L. M. (Eds). (2022). *Archaeologies of Indigenous presence*. University Press of Florida.

Sealey, D. B., & Lussier, A. S. (1975). *The Métis: Canada's forgotten people*. Manitoba Metis Federation Press.

Smith, C., & Wobst, H. M. (2004). *Indigenous archaeologies: Decolonizing theory and practice*. Routledge.

Supernant, K. (2018). Reconciling the past for the future: The next 50 years of Canadian archaeology in the post-TRC era. *Canadian Journal of Archaeology, 42*(1), 144–163. https://www.jstor.org/stable/44878258

Trinks, I., Hinterleitner, A., Neubauer, W., Nau, E., Löcker, K., Wallner, M., Gabler, M., Filzwieser, R., Wilding, J., Schiel, H., Jansa, V., Schneidhofer, P., Trausmuth, T., Sandici, V., Ruß, D., Flory, S., Kainz, J., Kucera, M., Vonklich, A., ... Seren, S. (2018). Large-area high-resolution ground-penetrating radar measurements for archaeological prospection. *Archaeological Prospection, 25*(3), 171–195. https://doi.org/10.1002/arp.1599

Twiss, K. (2019). *The archaeology of food: Identity, politics, and ideology in the prehistoric and historic past*. Cambridge University Press.

Van Kirk, S. (1980). *Many tender ties: Women in fur-trade society, 1670–1870*. University of Oklahoma Press.

Wadsworth, W. T. D., Supernant, K., & Kravchinsky, V. A. (2021). An integrated remote sensing approach to Métis archaeology in the Canadian Prairies. *Archaeological Prospection, 28*(3), 321–337. https://doi.org/10.1002/arp.1813

Wambold, D. (2021). *Beyond the beads: The representation of Métis women in the archaeological record* [Master's thesis, University of Alberta].

Watkins, J. (2005). Through wary eyes: Indigenous perspectives on archaeology. *Annual Review of Anthropology, 34*, 429–449. https://doi.org/10.1146/annurev.anthro.34.081804.120540

Weekes, M. (1994). *The last buffalo hunter: As told to her by Norbert Welsh*. Fifth House Books.

Weinbender, K. D. (2003). *Petite ville: A spatial assessment of a Métis hivernant site* [Master's thesis, University of Saskatchewan]. http://hdl.handle.net/10388/etd-03042009-133642

Wildcat, M. (2018). Wahkohtowin in action. *Constitutional Forum, 27*(1). https://doi.org/10.21991/cf29370

· 7 ·

ON BEING ELSEWHERE TO STAY: REFLECTIONS ON MÉTIS RESPONSIBILITIES LIVING IN THE HOMELANDS OF OTHER PEOPLE

Robert L. A. Hancock

The ideas in this chapter emerge from my reflections on two experiences I had at events hosted in the 2010s by the Métis Nation of Greater Victoria (MNGV), a chartered community affiliated with the Métis Nation of British Columbia (MNBC). I have been thinking about, with, and through these experiences for a long time and until now have had some trepidation to write about them for a number of reasons: they engage with different aspects of Métis studies than those within which I am used to working, they touch on more personal aspects of my own experiences and those of my family, and they come close to connecting with topics and areas of current interest and contention and political and interpersonal conflicts in my wider circle of relations, friends, and community members. All the same, I recognize that addressing and analyzing these experiences here—in spite of my misgivings—is both important and timely, as over the past few years I have been asked questions that relate to these ideas by a number of students and community members. I have also recognized the importance and growing urgency of learning my own family's stories as the generation above me gets older.

The first experience was a conversation with another MNGV community member who was encouraging me to register for my MNBC harvesting permit. I initially demurred on the grounds that I was neither a hunter nor a fisher.

When the person persisted, insisting that it was essential for several reasons to increase the number of permit holders, I responded that it was pointless in any case because I did not have any territory to hunt on in British Columbia. The reply was that as Canadians we have a right to hunt anywhere on Crown land. I left the conversation feeling confused by this response, because I could not imagine going onto another nation's territory to hunt without their permission, no matter what status was assigned to that land by the Canadian government.

The second experience happened at an event hosted by MNGV at the University of Victoria. We did a round of introductions, and several people acknowledged that they lived on ləkʷəŋən or W̱SÁNEĆ territory. It came around to one community member, who began by talking about how tired they were about always having to start "our" events by talking about another nation. They expressed frustration that in what they perceived as a wholly and solely Métis space (in a Coast Salish-style building), they were expected to talk about anybody other than Métis people and topics. The Elder and the student who were facilitating the introductions both looked to me to reply, and I responded that while it was true that this was a Métis event, the fact was that we were on territory that belonged to other nations and that it was incumbent upon us to acknowledge this fact whenever we gathered.

I am not saying that these two illustrations are representative of the perspectives of the entire MNGV membership. At the same time, relatives and colleagues have shared similar experiences from other places outside the Métis homeland, which makes me recognize that I have a responsibility to address them as a way to open conversations with other folks who are dealing with the same issues. My initial conclusions fall into three general areas. The first is that focusing on our "right" as Métis people to be in other people's territories, rather than on our responsibilities that arise from being there, is a move based on weakness rather than strength. The second is that a reliance on Canada to recognize us and our rights brings with it certain problematic aspects (Coulthard, 2014), while the third is that to rely on outside recognition and downplay our own responsibilities denigrates the strength and power of Métis forms of relating, asking permission, and making commitments about our presence.

I have also been thinking through the connections that are formed among the ideas that arise in my reflections on these vignettes. There are the connections to my own story and to my family's stories about being away from the Métis homelands and in the homelands of the ləkʷəŋən for two generations now. There are connections to my earlier work in Métis studies, particularly on peoplehood (Hancock, 2021), that draws on the work of the Cherokee anthropologist Robert K. Thomas to think about the ways that relationships to a place or stories about the loss of relationships with a place can shape collective identities and understandings. What connects these areas is the importance of understanding our responsibilities (as individuals, as families, as communities, as a nation) not only with reference to our current contexts but also based on what has come before in both community and academic settings.

There are also connections with work that other scholars have been doing, in both Métis settings and anthropology. Métis examples include the essential work of Daniel Voth and Jessie Loyer on the problems that arise with claiming territory based on mere presence in the absence of other factors (2019), Stephen Mussell's analysis of the problems with emergent Métis claims to territory and rights west of the Rockies (2020, 2021), and the work discussing Métis kinship and connections between individuals and families as webs or networks, drawing on the analyses of Nicole St-Onge and Carolyn Podruchny (2012), or as kinscapes, based on the analyses of Brenda Macdougall (2021). The key anthropological example is drawn from the work of Michael Asch, an academic Elder and one of my most important mentors; the title of this chapter (originally suggested by David Parent) is an homage to Asch's *On Being Here to Stay* (2014), the writing and teaching of which has allowed me to enter into a dialogue with him about what it means to have stronger connections in somebody else's homelands than those that are (ostensibly) my own.

From my reading of these other works, two key questions arise. The first centers on how we can make and maintain relations as we move around, which is connected to processes of remaking and revitalizing kinship ties and practices. The second focuses on the changes that arise when colonial boundaries are considered, and what it means to consider mobility before, after, and beyond the state.

Monkmans inləkʷəŋən Territory

I was born and raised in ləkʷəŋən territory to parents who were also born there. On my father's side I am English Canadian and through my paternal grandmother I am descended from a family who first arrived in ləkʷəŋən territory in the 1860s. On my mother's side I am Métis; my maternal grandfather, George "Buster" Monkman, came to Victoria with my grandmother Rita (who was of Swiss-German ancestry) during World War II. He was born in Treaty 8 territory to Alex and Louisa (née Tate) and raised on a homestead at Cutbank Lake near Lake Saskatoon but left the farm at the beginning of the Depression. From what I have learned about his departure, it was a result of both push factors (his eldest brother's growing family meant that there was not enough food to go around, and there was also some violence in the family) and pull factors (hope and a need for employment). There is a period of about eight years where we know very little about where he was or what he was doing before he ended up in Vancouver in 1939 or 1940; we have at least one letter he sent to his mother, any others he may have sent have been lost. Louisa's family were the Tates from Edmonton, which introduces another aspect of mobility, related to class and operating in both directions, from the late nineteenth century through the twentieth century.

According to our genealogical records, my generation was the first in my mother's family to be born in the same place our parents were born, going back to the middle of the nineteenth century. Based on baptismal and marriage certificates, my direct Métis ancestors appear to have already been on their way west out of Red River by about 1868. I am learning from my conversations with other relations and colleagues that these experiences were not all that uncommon among Métis families during the middle part of the twentieth century. We can see evidence of not only physical mobility but also class mobility, each connected in its own way with military service and wage labor, reinforcing Chris Andersen's reminder of the importance of engaging this period in a meaningful way for understanding current Métis situations and experiences rather than focusing solely on the nineteenth century (2014, p. 629).

These histories of mobility and its causes have significant implications for our own and our families' current sense of place. This can be seen in the idea of "home," for people who have moved every generation (and/or multiple times during their lives). It can also be observed in the concept of "the homeland(s)," for people whose families last lived there a long time ago and have lived elsewhere far longer than their ancestors lived there; we have to engage with the impact and implications of centering the homeland(s) in understandings of Métis belonging and identity and ask if we assume that people are less Métis or not Métis at all because they do not live there or do not want or are not able to live there. Finally, it can be perceived in the question of how our ancestors would recognize us when we live in places other than they did, and therefore in the linked question of what constitutes the "essential" aspects of being Métis and how these can be lived elsewhere; I have been focusing on family and relationships through the concept of wahkohtowin (Hancock, 2017) and on responsibilities to all beings, human and other-than-human, wherever I am, drawing on the work of Elmer Ghostkeeper (2007), Zoe Todd (2017), and Jennifer Adese (2014). Taken together, all these aspects help point the ways toward Métis models of decolonization and resurgence, recognizing that mobility is both a historical and current fact that needs to be addressed in any work we do.

Moving Ahead

Based on these analyses and experiences, my key motivating question when considering my presence in ləkʷəŋən territory has become a consideration of what we need to do as Métis people to be elsewhere in ways that respect our own teachings and values and those of the people on whose lands we are living. This is an issue for all Métis people, not just those of us who live away from the homelands, as it is inevitable that we have relatives who have been or are living elsewhere or that we will find ourselves travelling through other people's territories for longer or shorter periods of time even if we do not end up settling there. In thinking through this question, I have drawn a key insight from the James Bay Cree scholar and administrator Ruth Young, who has demonstrated that our theoretical and methodological approaches as Indigenous researchers depend both on who we are and where we are; that is, that we need to find a way to work that respects both our own ways of knowing and being and those of the people on whose lands we live and work (2022, p. 9).

I am thinking through this in two ways. The first comes from reflecting on the common talk in Métis spaces about being good hosts and wondering why we do not speak as much about the necessity of being good guests; this is connected with the realization that without guests there can be no hosts. The second comes from teachings shared by ləkʷəŋən Elder Skip Dick about how to be in this place, starting with demonstrating respect for the local people as the foundation for practicing our own ways. I have never heard him say that other people should not practice their own ways; instead, he emphasizes the importance of holding onto their own practices and teachings so that their relatives do not think that the ləkʷəŋən are trying to make them into ləkʷəŋən people and so that others can share their ways with him if he ever travels to their territories.

I am coming to understand that addressing these issues requires an expansive, intentional, and conscientious approach in at least three directions. First, it means recognizing and analyzing the historical and contemporary colonial policies and practices that make it possible for us as Métis people to be in other people's territories without following proper protocols, either ours or theirs. Second, it requires a serious reconsideration of our assumptions and worries about what it means to be here in other people's territories and what might happen if we try to be here differently. If we accept, as I do, that the legitimacy of everything we do is predicated on good relations, then we have more work to do in a place where we do not already have relatives. This requires letting go of our desire for a space where we can be dominant and set the rules unilaterally and instead accepting a place where we have to be vulnerable and getting past the idea that our mere presence in a place is grounds enough to demand respect from the people who are already there. The need for this practice is especially acute if we are not willing or able to leave other people's territory, or if there is not an obvious place for us to "return," in which case we need to figure out how to be there legitimately, first on their terms and only then on our own.

Finally, addressing this issue is both a matter of accountability and an opportunity for us as Métis people to renew and re-engage with knowledge about and practice of protocols around travelling, visiting, and being in other people's places ethically and legitimately. Mussell (2020) expresses this idea particularly powerfully:

> What is required is a transformation of our relationships. We must focus our time, resources and energy on revitalizing and reclaiming our own law and legal traditions and understanding how our ancestors related to and interacted with peoples whose lands we settled on. We must work with First Nations to establish legal, economic and kinship relations—some might say *treaties*—in ways which honour and strengthen their laws and legal traditions, uphold our own, and provide us with legally and morally defensible access to resources on their lands and within their waters with their consent. (p. 3)

Mussell outlines a concrete approach and a compelling rationale that reflects both internal and external priorities and advantages in terms of strengthening our own understandings of Métis practices and concepts and of improving our relationships with the people on whose territories we are living by ensuring that our goals are not only aligned with but actively support their goals.

This discussion brings me back to the vignettes with which I opened the chapter and the ways that my reflection on them have motivated and shaped my work with my own family. I am committed to addressing the obligations that arise when we interrogate the stories about how we came to be in ləkʷəŋən territory and what it means to want to stay here. I am also envisioning the other stories that can be told about being here and about legitimizing our presence, particularly those that will reduce our appeals to Canadian identity and authority to validate our presence here. This means both coming to a better understanding of how and why my family came to be here, of how our story connects with other Métis families' experiences of mobility and residence outside the homelands, and of how those of us in this situation can connect with one another and with people in the homelands to bring back Métis practices of diplomacy and permission-seeking in conjunction with wider projects of Métis resurgence.

Acknowledgments

I have had the opportunity to share earlier versions of the ideas in this chapter at the Indigenous Research Workshop hosted by the Centre for Indigenous Research and Community-Led Engagement at the University of Victoria, at the Mawachihitotaak online conference, and at the Indigenous Relationality Workshop organized by the Prairie Indigenous Relationality Network at the Prairie Political Science Association in Banff. I am grateful for the feedback and suggestions offered in each of these settings and in individual conversations with Heidi Stark, Phil Henderson, Stacie Swain, David Parent, Adam Gaudry, Elaine Alexie, Matt Wildcat, and Daniel Voth.

References

Adese, J. (2014). Spirit gifting: Ecological knowing in Métis life narratives. *Decolonization: Indigeneity, Education, and Society*, 3(3), 48–66. https://jps.library.utoronto.ca/index.php/des/article/view/22191

Andersen, C. (2014). More than the sum of our rebellions: Métis histories beyond Batoche. *Ethnohistory*, 61(4), 619–633. https://doi.org/10.1215/00141801-2717795

Asch, M. (2014). *On being here to stay: Treaties and Aboriginal rights in Canada*. University of Toronto Press.

Coulthard, G. S. (2014). *Red skin, white masks: Rejecting the colonial politics of recognition*. University of Minnesota Press.

Ghostkeeper, E. (2007). *Spirit gifting: The concept of spiritual exchange*. Writing on Stone Press.

Hancock, R. L. A. (2021). The power of peoplehood: Reimagining Métis relationships, research, and responsibilities. In J. Adese & C. Andersen (Eds.), *A people and a nation: New directions in contemporary Métis studies* (pp. 51–77). UBC Press.

Hancock, R. L. A. (2017). "We know who our relatives are": Métis identities in historical, political, and legal contexts. In J. Carrière & C. Richardson (Eds.), *Calling our families home: Métis peoples' experiences with child welfare* (pp. 9–30). J Charlton.

Macdougall, B. (2021). How we know who we are: Historical literacy, kinscapes, and defining a people. In N. Kermoal & C. Andersen (Eds.), Daniels v. Canada: *In and beyond the courts*, (pp. 233–267). University of Manitoba Press.

Mussell, S. (2020). Do Métis have rights in British Columbia? Let our Métis people be heard in a good way. Yellowhead Institute Policy Brief 78. https://yellowheadinstitute.org/2020/10/22/do-metis-have-rights-in-british-columbia-let-our-metis-people-be-heard-in-a-good-way/

Mussell, S. (2021). In defence of the integrity of our nation: Métis colonialism west of the Rocky Mountains. Yellowhead Institute Policy Brief 94. https://yellowheadinstitute.org/2021/04/06/in-defence-of-the-integrity-of-our-nation-metis-colonialism-west-of-the-rocky-mountains/

St-Onge, N., & Podruchny, C. (2012). Scuttling along a spider's web: Mobility and kinship in Metis ethnogenesis. In N. St-Onge, C. Podruchny, & B. Macdougall (Eds.), *Contours of a people: Metis family, mobility, and history* (pp. 59–92). University of Oklahoma Press.

Todd, Z. (2017). From a fishy place: Tending to water violations in amiskwasi wâskahikan and Treaty 6 territory. *Afterall: A Journal of Arts, Context, and Enquiry, 43*, 102–107. https://www.journals.uchicago.edu/doi/full/10.1086/692559

Voth, D., & Loyer, J. (2019). Why Calgary isn't Métis territory: Jigging towards an ethic of reciprocal visiting. In G. Starblanket & D. Long, with O. P. Dickason (Eds.), *Visions of the heart: Issues involving Indigenous peoples in Canada* (5th ed., pp. 106–125). Oxford University Press.

Young, R. (2022). *"Know when to hold 'em, know when to fold 'em": Navigating the more-than-dual roles of Indigenous leadership in post-secondary colonial institutions* [Master's thesis, University of Victoria]. http://hdl.handle.net/1828/13922

· 8 ·

"IT'S VERY DIFFERENT WALKING IN TWO WORLDS AS A MÉTIS PERSON": IDENTITY, COMMUNITY, CULTURE AND CONNECTIONS AS DETERMINANTS OF THE HEALTH AND WELLBEING OF MÉTIS PEOPLES

Heather Foulds, Jamie LaFleur and Leah Ferguson

Author Biographies

Heather Foulds

Heather Foulds, PhD (she/her/hers), is a member of Métis Nation–Saskatchewan and Saskatoon Métis Local 126, and descends from the Métis communities of Bresaylor and Langmeade, Saskatchewan. She is an Associate Professor in the College of Kinesiology at the University of Saskatchewan and the Heart and Stroke/CIHR Indigenous Early Career Women's Heart and Brain Health Chair. She is Co-Scientific Director of the mamawiikikayaahk (Healing Together) Métis Research Network of the Saskatchewan Network Environment for Indigenous Health Research. Her research partners with Métis communities to evaluate the importance of cultural connections, identity, and social support as determinants of cardiovascular disease for Métis people and how Métis dancing can improve health and wellbeing.

Jamie LaFleur

Jamie LaFleur is a Rock Cree woman from Lac La Ronge Indian Band and the daughter of a proud Métis man from Beauval, Saskatchewan. She has an honors degree in anthropology specializing in medical anthropology and is now in her second year of an MSc in epidemiology and community health at the University of Saskatchewan College of Medicine. Over the course of her undergraduate work, she completed four study abroad programs in Norway, Thailand, Ukraine, and South Africa, all for health studies. Her master's thesis is part of the Pathways to Health Equity for Indigenous Peoples Initiative in Canada. She is also a sponsored Ironman triathlete.

Leah Ferguson

Leah Ferguson, PhD (she/her/hers), is a member of the Métis Nation–Saskatchewan and Saskatoon Métis Local 126. She is an Associate Professor in the College of Kinesiology at the University of Saskatchewan and Co-Scientific Director of the mamawiikikayaahk (Healing Together) Métis Research Network of the Saskatchewan Network Environment for Indigenous Health Research. She is committed to community and scholarly engagement with Indigenous people, and she works with Indigenous youth, girls, women, athletes, and community members to collaboratively enhance holistic wellness. Her research is rooted in building relationships, and she prioritizes community members' voices to guide the direction of her research.

Introduction

This chapter surveys the quantitative and qualitative research exploring the importance of identity, community, and culture for physical activity and the health and wellbeing of Métis people through evaluating exercise associations with cultural connectedness and social support and conversational interviews exploring relations of Métis identity, community, and connections with health and wellbeing. Métis meeting musculoskeletal exercise guidelines reported greater social support, and Métis who relocated from home communities were more likely to meet musculoskeletal exercise guidelines. Less physically active Métis reported stronger connections to cultural traditions and spirituality. Métis experiencing greater discrimination or having experienced foster care or residential school participated in more traditional activities. Thematic analysis of qualitative data identified six important aspects of health and wellbeing for Métis peoples: (1) the Métis person: "I have a lot to learn about myself and my culture, where I come from"; (2) balancing the Métis duality: "on the phone I have my white voice"; (3) the Métis community as a pillar of health: "Community, I think is the foundation that health and wellness have to be built on"; (4) the Métis diet and health outcomes: "Food sovereignty ... it's a perfect example of capital racism"; (5) the Métis environment and land connection: "The water is like a route home ... that connection actually makes me walk more"; and (6) Métis ceremony and its connection to Métis wellbeing: "Wearing that sash makes you feel more strength on your shoulders (...) like a support system on your back." Identity, community, and cultural connections, including foods and land, influence Métis people's health and wellbeing.

Métis peoples are a distinct Indigenous nation with a unique history, culture, language, and identity (Andersen, 2014; Dorion & Préfontaine, 2003; Gaudry, 2018; Macdougall, 2017). The culture and spirituality practices of Métis people reflect the importance of community, environment, and religion (Andersen, 2014; Dorion & Préfontaine, 2003; Gaudry, 2018; Macdougall, 2017). Traditionally, health and wellbeing were tied to extended kinship networks, recognizing an understanding of mutual responsibility across Métis kinship, society, and community (Macdougall, 2017). Métis worldviews, knowledge, perspectives, and voices support Métis people and communities to thrive, while fragmentation and the silencing of Métis people and communities by colonization and racism have led to substantive health disparities among them (Greenwood et al., 2018; Mitrou et al., 2014; Wilson & Macdonald, 2010). Cultural components of wellbeing, including identity, attitudes, and acculturation, can mediate the poorer health and quality of life resulting from historical traumas disconnecting Métis people from their traditional culture, values, and beliefs (Barton et al., 2005; Craib et al., 2009; Lavallée, 2007, Walters & Simoni, 2002). Social experiences are also known to impact health and wellbeing, including globalization, migration, colonization, loss of culture and language, disconnection from land, socioeconomic inequalities, and connectivity deficits (King et al., 2009).

Métis-specific experiences of health and wellbeing, including sociopolitical and historical experiences, differ from experiences of First Nation and Inuit peoples; however, distinct health determinants of Métis people are rarely recognized (Dorion & Préfontaine, 2003; Gaudry, 2018). While health inequities among Métis people may be similar to that of First Nations,

Métis-specific health experiences are poorly understood (Andersen, 2016; Foulds et al., 2013, Monchalin & Monchalin, 2018; Sheppard et al., 2017). Cultural and social determinants of health and wellbeing among Indigenous peoples are being recognized (Roh et al., 2015; Walters & Simoni, 2002). Specific to Métis people, emerging determinants of health and wellbeing may also include community and family support, the Michif language, Métis cultural identity, and experiences with and disruptions of connections with individuals, community, and the environment.

This chapter outlines key findings from recent studies exploring Métis-specific cultural and social determinants of health and wellbeing. It first evaluates the importance of identity and cultural connectedness in physical activity specifically and health and wellbeing more broadly. Second, the importance of community for Métis people is discussed in relation to physical activity behaviors and health and wellbeing. The importance of connections, including challenges to connections caused by experiences of discrimination and personal and family histories of residential school and foster care, are explored in relation to physical activity. Connections with culture and community in the form of food and environment are then further explored in relation to Métis health and wellbeing.

Research Approaches

As previously reported (Ironside et al., 2020, 2021), under the direction of community advisors including Indigenous undergraduate and graduate students, staff, faculty, and an Elder, selected by partnering with Indigenous groups (i.e., the Indigenous Graduate Student Association, the Indigenous Student Achievement Program, staff at the Aboriginal Students' Centre, and other Indigenous groups at the University of Saskatchewan), an online survey was developed, received institutional and community advisory ethics approval, and was administered to evaluate associations of cultural connectedness and social support with physical activity among Indigenous people at the University of Saskatchewan, including 41 Métis people (30 women, 11 men) (Ironside et al., 2020, 2021). Cultural connectedness was assessed through the general population multigroup ethnic identity measure (Brown et al., 2014; Herrington et al., 2016; Phinney, 1992) and the Indigenous-specific cultural connectedness Scale (Snowshoe et al., 2015, 2017). Multiple social determinants were assessed, as previously described (Ironside et al., 2021), through the social support index (Distelberg et al., 2014) and family support questionnaire (Wang et al., 2015), and community designed and identified questions around family and personal attendance at residential school, family and personal foster care placements, participant's home community, and discrimination experiences (Edwards & Cunningham, 2013; Williams, 1999). Physical activity assessment included weekly moderate-to-vigorous physical activity (MVPA) summed from the Godin-Shephard leisure time exercise questionnaire (Godin & Shephard, 1985), meeting twice weekly musculoskeletal exercise (MSK) guidelines (Ross et al., 2020), and participation in traditional activities (Ironside et al., 2020, 2021).

In partnership with Saskatoon Métis Local 126 and four Métis Community Advisors from the University of Saskatchewan, a qualitative study approved by both community and university ethics processes with 20 Métis adults (10 men, 10 women) was carried out; it included conversational group and individual interviews followed by a reflexive photovoice exercise (Phoenix, 2010) and a second "photo elicitation" (Kovach, 2009) conversational interview to gain understanding of the importance of cultural connectedness and social support for the health and wellbeing of Métis adults. Questions in the first conversational interview asked about participants' experiences with social support and health (e.g., *How might social support be related to health and wellbeing?*). Questions around culture and health were then asked, beginning with general thoughts (e.g., *How might culture be related to health and wellbeing?*) and moving to more specific thoughts (e.g., *What aspects of Métis culture influence or could influence your health and wellbeing?*). The final questions focused on identity and culture in relation to health (e.g., *How is your identity as a Métis person and your participation in Métis culture related to your health and wellbeing?*). The second interview engaged dialogue around participants' photographs (e.g., *What does this photograph tell about your experiences of culture and/or social support and your health and wellbeing?*). Reflexive thematic analysis (Charmaz, 2006; Creswell, 2014) identified six themes describing the importance of culture and social support in the health and wellbeing of Métis people.

Identity

Connections to culture and important aspects of identity for Métis people were similar among Métis reporting high and low MVPA (Figure 1A) and meeting or not meeting MSK guidelines (Figure 1B) when evaluated using a general population questionnaire. Conversely, as assessed using an Indigenous-specific cultural connectedness questionnaire, Métis reporting lower MVPA reported greater connections to cultural traditions and spirituality though similar identity and overall cultural connectedness (Figure 1C) to those reporting higher MVPA. Cultural connections were similar among Métis meeting and not meeting MSK guidelines (Figure 1D).

The first theme identified through interviews and photovoice explorations of Métis-specific determinants of health and wellness focused on the Métis person: "I have a lot to learn about myself and my culture, where I come

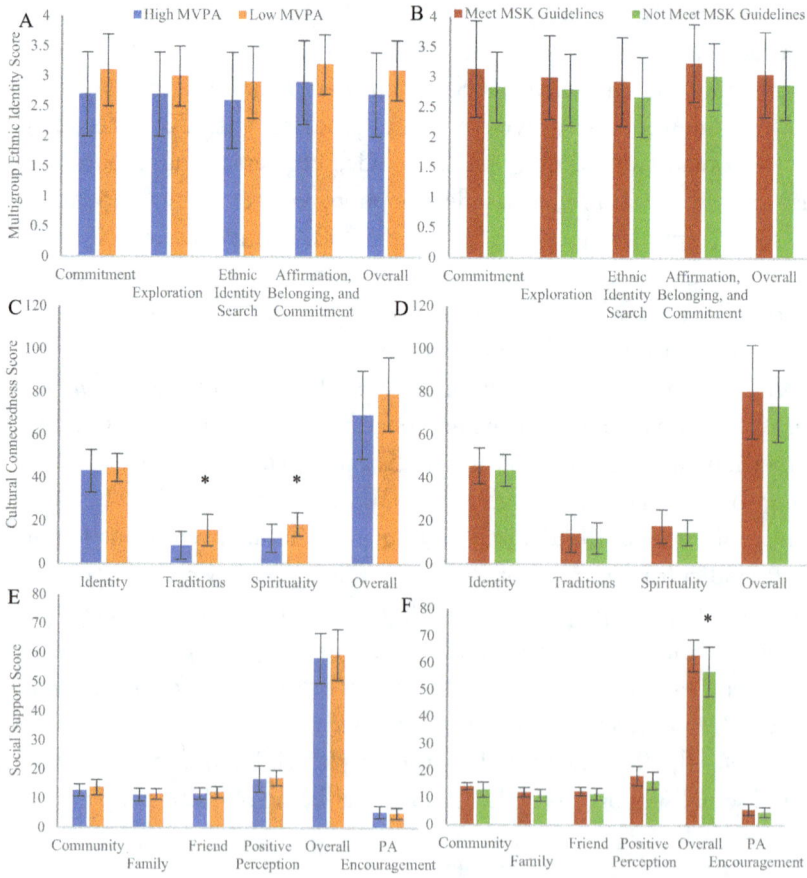

Figure 1: Cultural connections as measured by Multigroup Ethnic Identity Measure (A and B) and Cultural Connectedness Scale (C and D), and community support as measured by Social Support Index and family support of physical activity (PA) questions (E and F) in relation to moderate-to-vigorous physical activity (MVPA; A, C and E) and meeting twice weekly musculoskeletal (MSK) exercise guidelines (B, D and F) among Metis adults at the University of Saskatchewan. MVPA divided at group median. Asterisk (*) indicates significant difference by physical activity at p<0.05.

from." In recognizing Métis identity as an important determinant of health and wellbeing, different aspects of Métis identity and the exploration and recognition of these aspects of identity were discussed. "Culture as self-discovery" was an important component of developing Métis identity, as articulated in a quote by participant Marlin Legare:[1] "Culture is identity and without identity, the brain is just wired to fall apart." Another aspect of Métis identity was "tracing family histories and lineages," as described by Kurt: "I'm excited to find out (...) where my ancestors came from and what they had to do and what they had to fight for." The third component of Métis identity was articulated around "actively 'being' Métis" and was well captured by Kurt noting that "finding out how strong Métis people actually are, it makes you, as a Métis person, feel more safe." Métis identity was further elaborated and articulated through photos shared in these discussions, as presented in Figure 2.

Balancing the Métis duality: "On the phone I have my white voice" was the second theme generated to understand Métis-specific determinants of health and wellbeing and further described through photographs from participants, as presented in Figure 2. Participants discussing this theme shared stories around their experiences and challenges in positioning themselves and societal expectations around their identity and appearance. A sub-theme "Reconciling non-Indigenous appearances and colorism discrimination" was well articulated by Danielle: "It was really difficult to reconcile my Métis identity with the German last name and a fair-skin body." A second sub-theme focused on "Feeling isolated due to having dual cultural backgrounds," with participants discussing experiences of not fitting in to either Indigenous spaces and colonized or European spaces or both. Experiences of racism were identified by Métis people, including the challenges of identifying as Métis while experiencing societal stereotypes of Indigenous peoples and the options of staying under the radar and passing as white in some spaces, despite the discomfort in not fully acknowledging one's identity. These experiences were well articulated by Desiree: "We were born with racism. We were told to hate our own kind our own people. We were told they were all drunks and druggies and that kind of thing." The final sub-theme that emerged in balancing dualities of Métis identity focused around "the politics of identity." In many colonized spaces, including the University of Saskatchewan, the representation of Indigenous peoples, knowledge, and cultures and the outward Indigenization initiatives primarily focus on First Nations peoples and cultures, leaving Métis feeling excluded and once again struggling to fit into either Indigenous or colonized or European spaces. Marlin Legare succinctly articulated this experience: "I really didn't find much Métis representation when I was there."

A The Metis Person: "I have a lot to learn about myself and my culture, where I come from"
'I think I would've been a really, really happy child if I had gotten to do jigging and fiddling in a context that was "happy Metis"' - Caroline

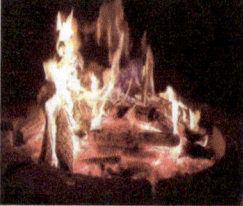 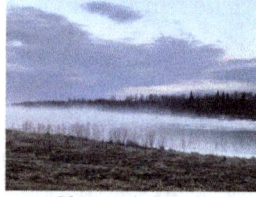 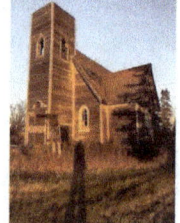

Photo credit Adam Dyck   *Photo credit Russell*   *Photo credit Susan Shacter*

B Balancing the Metis Duality: "on the phone I have my white voice"
"I'm Indigenous, but my skin is white and I have green eyes" - Kate Boyer

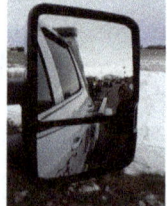 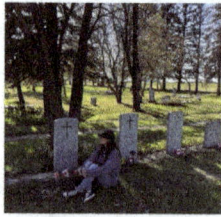 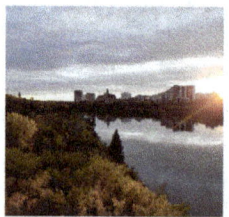

Photo credit Joselyn   *Photo credit Caroline*   *Photo credit Danielle*

C The Metis Community as a Pillar of Health: "Community, I think is the foundation that health and wellness have to be built on"
"So, that community part, I think, Is really essential for me. For me, as far as health and wellbeing going, and if I'm blocking that, then I feel isolated" - Steve Fraser

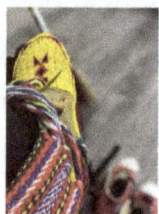 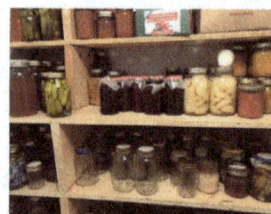 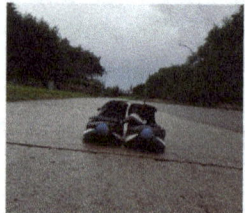

Photo credit Kate Boyer   *Photo credit Randi*   *Photo credit Adam Dyck*

Figure 2: Photovoice images describing themes of 1) The Metis Person (A); 2) Balancing the Metis Duality (B); and 3) The Metis Community as a Pillar of Health (C) exploring the importance of cultural connectedness and social support in the health of Metis Peoples.

Community

Social support can be obtained from many sources, including family, friends, and community, and people are influenced by perceptions of available sources of support. Social supports, including community, family, friends, a positive perception of support, and overall social support, along with family support of physical activity, were similar among Métis who reported higher and lower weekly MVPA (Figure 1E). Though specific dimensions of social support were similar between Métis meeting and not meeting weekly MSK guidelines, overall social support was greater among those who met those guidelines (Figure 1F).

Métis who come from northern home communities reported similar MVPA (Figure 3A) as those coming from home communities that they considered southern. Similarly, Métis from rural home communities reported MVPA similar to Métis from urban home communities (Figure 3A). Reported MVPA was also similar among Métis who had and had not relocated from their home communities (Figure 3A). The proportion of Métis meeting MSK guidelines was similar among Métis from northern and southern home communities and those from urban and rural home communities (Figure 3B). A greater proportion of Métis who had left their home communities reported meeting MSK guidelines than those who had not (Figure 3B). Looking more closely at Métis experiences of leaving home communities in relation to physical activity, individuals who had relocated from home communities reported greater connections to Métis identity, traditions, spirituality, and overall cultural connectedness, as measured by an Indigenous-specific cultural connectedness questionnaire.

Métis-specific determinants of health and wellbeing identified in conversations with Métis peoples included the Métis community as a pillar of health: "Community, I think is the foundation that health and wellness have to be built on." In recognizing community as a determinant of health and wellbeing, Métis people shared experiences and importance of different aspects of community, including "Métis social events." These social events and their importance are highlighted by a quote from Marlin Legare: "At jigging events (...) you're going to have Elders there. You're going to have maybe even relatives you didn't even know about, so to be able to get that connection, get involved in that (...) [is] something I'm actively pursuing." Discussions around the importance of community for the health and wellbeing of Métis adults also identified "Métis social connections" as an important component of community. These discussions shared stories and experiences in supporting other Métis in the community, working together on initiatives, and how children were supported and protected by the whole community. An example of these community social connections was articulated by Susan:

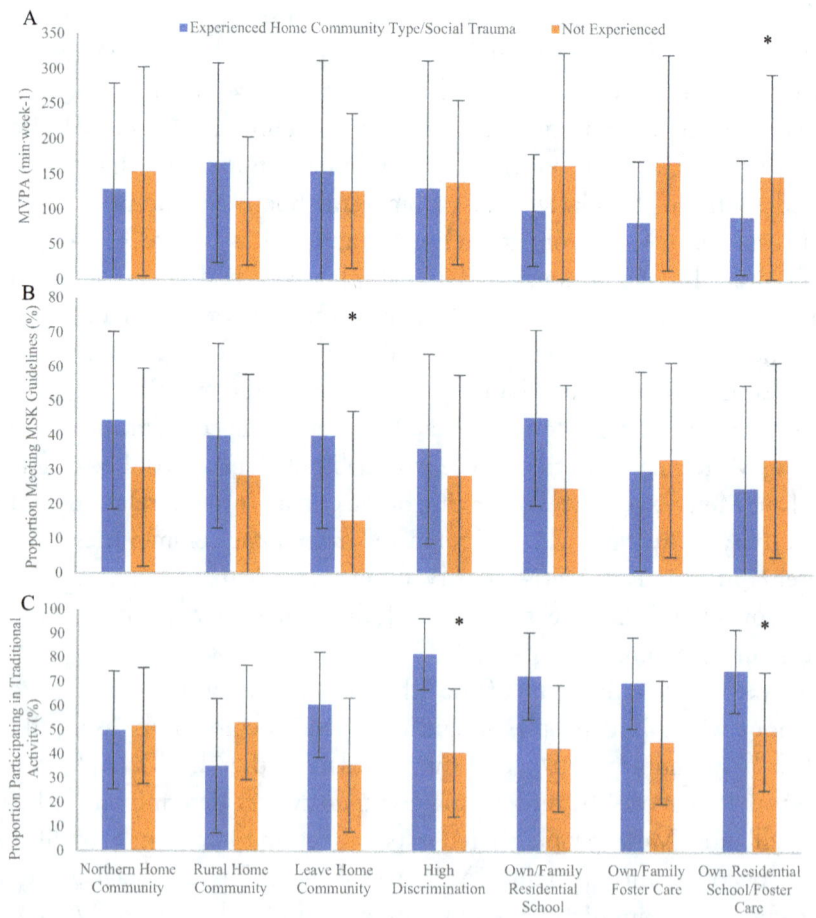

Figure 3: Weekly moderate-to-vigorous physical activity (MVPA; A), the proportion of participants meeting twice weekly musculoskeletal (MSK) exercise guidelines (B) and the proportion of participants participating in traditional activity (C) among Metis adults at the University of Saskatchewan by experiences of social factors including home residence type, discrimination, and personal or family residential school attendance and foster care placements. Asterisk (*) indicates significant difference between experienced vs. not at p<0.05.

All the people in the community would hunt together, and my dad was one who would cut up all the meat.(...) It was a time of celebration and it was a time of the harvest season.(...) If somebody didn't get an animal, we shared our meat with them. So everybody went home with meat and our freezers were stocked for the winter, and it was just a fun time.

In understanding the importance of Métis community for health and wellbeing, additional understandings of the importance of "Métis in sport" emerged, with participants sharing stories and experiences of how they use sport as a way to become stronger community members and the ways communities support them through sport. Trent described the experience of community through sport as follows:

Everybody knows you. So when there's volleyball (...) they will drive two and a half hours, and half of a community, to watch you do that, or they'll drive out to the middle of nowhere to a ranch to watch you participate in an equine discipline, and that's the kind of community I have behind me.

These important discussions were enriched through sharing of photographs; see examples in Figure 2.

Connections

Weekly MVPA was similar between Métis who faced high versus low or moderate discrimination and those reporting personal or family experiences at residential schools or personal or family experiences in foster care (Figure 3A). Similar proportions of Métis reported meeting weekly MSK guidelines (Figure 3B) among Métis facing high versus low or moderate discrimination and Métis with personal or family experiences in residential schools or in foster care. Among Métis with personal experiences in residential school or foster care, weekly MVPA was lower than among Métis without those experiences (Figure 3A), though similar proportions of Métis with and without personal residential school or foster care experiences met MSK guidelines.

Métis participation in traditional activities was similar among Métis from northern and southern home communities, rural and urban home communities, and among Métis who had and had not left their home communities (Figure 3C). Similarly, the proportions of Métis participating in traditional activities were similar among Métis with and without personal or family experience in residential schools or in foster care. A greater proportion of Métis who reported facing high discrimination participated in traditional activities than Métis experiencing low or moderate discrimination. Similarly, Métis who had personally attended residential schools or been placed in foster care were more likely to participate in traditional activities than Métis without these personal experiences. Participation in traditional activities among Métis was also associated with connections to culture, where Métis who participate in traditional activities reported greater connections to Métis identity, traditions, spirituality, and overall cultural connectedness, as measured with an Indigenous-specific questionnaire.

The Métis diet and health outcomes: "Food sovereignty ... it's a perfect example of capital racism" was identified as an important component of health and wellbeing specific to Métis people. In understanding the importance of foods and diet for Métis health and wellbeing, the subtheme "Food as culture" discussed the sharing of foods, the harvested and homegrown foods Métis people prioritized, and the disruption of culture through food with the processed foods now readily available. This disruption of culture through food was clearly articulated by Adam Dyck: "Processed food being brought over, and there was that loss of culture in terms of food preparation." This conflict between food sources was further articulated in the subtheme of "Traditional vs. western nutrition" and clearly articulated by Russell: "The food system in North America is failing us." A final subtheme around Métis foods focused on "Métis determinants of health" and included discussions around the enjoyment of cooking and food preparation and the feelings of connections to one's community that are achieved through food, even when one is physically away from community. These discussions are represented by the following remark by Joselyn: "Last bowl of soup, but it was so, so good, and it reminded me of home and being surrounded by the people who cared for me." These discussions of the importance of food in health and wellbeing were further elaborated through discussions and the sharing of photographs, some of which appear in Figure 4.

The fifth theme identified in understanding Métis-specific determinants of health and wellbeing was the Métis environment and land connection: "The water is like a route home ... that connection actually makes me walk more," which focused on the importance of finding connections to land and the environment regardless of where one is. Métis peoples shared stories and experiences of their need to find spaces on the land to escape western, colonized lifestyles, feeling recharged on the lands and connections to community through the land, which were augmented by photographs (see Figure 4). The connections to land in relation to health and wellbeing are described by Danielle as

A The Metis Diet and Health Outcomes: "Food sovereignty…it's a perfect example of capital racism"
"The people you are with effect how you eat…I never realized how much that impacted my overall health - Desiree

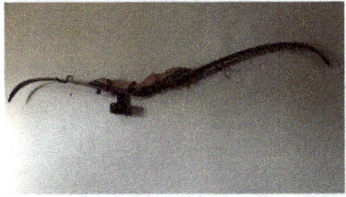 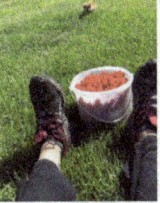 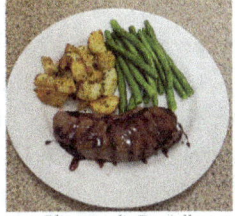

Photo credit Marlin Legare   *Photo credit Randi*   *Photo credit Danielle*

B The Metis Environment and Land Connection: "The water is like a route home…that connection actually makes me walk more"
"Out in the forest…it's actually so humbling and I feel like to just resets you"- Joselyn

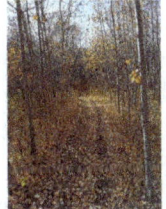 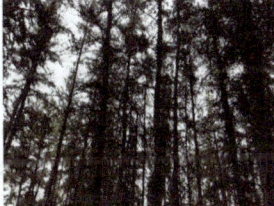 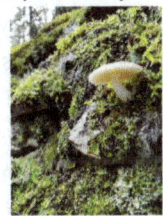

Photo credit Justin Norton   *Photo credit Marlin Legare*   *Photo credit Joselyn*

C Metis Ceremony and its Connection to Metis Wellbeing: "Wearing that sash makes you feel more strength on your shoulders… like a support system on your back"
"My culture and my jigging and my language – the food and everything. It's sometimes about listening"- Kurt

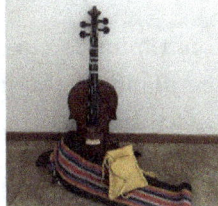 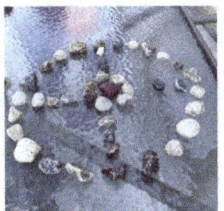 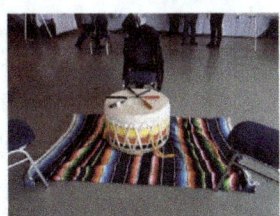

Photo credit Marlin Legare   *Photo credit Desiree McCarthy*   *Photo credit Steve Fraser*

Figure 4: Photovoice images describing themes of 1) The Metis Diet and Health Outcomes (A); 2) The Metis Environment and Land Connections (B); and 3) Metis Ceremony and its Connection to Metis Wellbeing (C) exploring the importance of cultural connectedness and social support in the health of Metis Peoples.

follows: "There's a medicine element to it too … belonging and support that comes from the land itself." Participants described finding land both within the city and beyond urban spaces; finding these places was important to health and wellbeing, as Kate Boyer put it: "Everybody has a connection to nature in some way … the nature that's around there is comforting to them."

The final theme in understanding Métis-specific determinants of health and wellbeing was Métis ceremony and its connection to Métis wellbeing: "Wearing that sash makes you feel more strength on your shoulders ... like a support system on your back," which included discussions of how learning about culture, traditions, language, and ceremony specific to Métis people brings health and wellbeing. Tyler identified this importance as follows: "Learning about the purpose behind [ceremonies] and how they came to be, that's huge. It's like a big revelation to me. Makes me understand my background more, and having that connection to your background is so vital." These discussions were supported by photos (see Figure 4).

Reflections

A sense of belonging is known to be a strong health determinant for Indigenous peoples in Canada (Richmond et al., 2007). Better overall social supports, suggesting a stronger sense of belonging among community, family, and friends, are linked to a greater likelihood of meeting weekly MSK guidelines among Métis. Those who have left their home communities may seek other avenues of health and wellbeing to augment these connections, such as engaging in exercise. Social support provides opportunities to overcome barriers to physical activity and health and wellbeing and provides increased enjoyment and motivation (Allender et al., 2006, Kahn et al., 2002).

Physical activity patterns of Métis who experience discrimination or have personal experiences in residential schools or foster care highlight the interconnectedness of culture, identity, physical activities, and the role of physical activity in supporting health and mediating trauma experiences. Links between separation from traditional beliefs, values, and culture with historic and ongoing traumas are well established among First Nations (Lavallée, 2007). These traumas have also been linked to increased health disparities and poorer quality of life (Barton et al., 2005; Craib et al. 2009). Lower weekly MVPA participation of Métis with personal experience in residential schools or foster care demonstrates these damaging impacts of residential schools and foster care on the health and wellbeing of Métis people. Engagement in culture (Walters & Simoni, 2002) and traditional physical activity (Lavallée, 2007) as coping methods for dealing with traumas, discrimination, and personal life experiences is well established among First Nations peoples. Métis people's experiences of this association of culture as a coping mechanism is supported by increased participation in traditional activities among Métis facing higher discrimination or with personal experiences of residential school and foster care. Conversely, Métis practicing traditional activities may face discrimination because of those practices. Overall, social experiences of discrimination, foster care, and residential schools influence traditional activity participation.

Métis culture, traditions, and identity have been heavily influenced by colonization and by both Protestant and Catholic churches (Logan, 2015). Spirituality, religion, and community structures among Métis are distinct from those among both First Nations and Euro-Canadians (Logan, 2015). Further, Métis individuals practice traditions, spirituality, and culture across a wide range of religions and beliefs, including aspects of First Nations and Euro-Canadian culture and Métis-specific culture, with many individuals practicing aspects of all these spiritualties (Giroux, 2016). Consequently, Métis culture and identity are more complex; they depend on individual and family identity acknowledgement, histories of hiding Métis identities, and the access and teachings individuals have had across multiple spiritualties (Richardson, 2004; Shore, 2001). Understanding connections of culture with physical activity and other health determinants and experiences among Métis people requires more detailed understandings of what culture means to them, how they practice and recognize their culture, and what aspects of culture are important and meaningful for health and wellbeing among Métis people.

Conclusions

Among Métis people, important determinants of health and wellbeing include having a well-developed sense of who one is and what it means to be Métis, along with having strong ties to community and connections with land, food, and culture. Having stronger connections, such as the combined supports of community, family, and friends, is associated with greater physical activity levels and health and wellbeing more broadly. Conversely, challenges to connections, such as residential school, foster care, and discrimination negatively influence physical activity levels and health and wellbeing more broadly. Métis people who are facing these challenges to connection may seek ways to maintain and reconnect with Métis culture, identity, and personhood by engaging with traditions, spirituality, and culture, including traditional activities.

Note

1 Participants used self-selected pseudonyms, their first names, or their full names, per their individual preference.

References

Allender, S., Cowburn, G., & Foster, C. (2006). Understanding participation in sport and physical activity among children and adults: A review of qualitative studies. *Health Education Research, 21*(6), 826–835. https://doi.org/10.1093/her/cyl063

Andersen, C. (2014). *"Métis": Race, recognition, and the struggle for Indigenous peoplehood.* UBC Press.

Andersen, C. (2016). The colonialism of Canada's Métis health population dynamics: Caught between bad data and no data at all. *Journal of Population Research, 33*(1), 67–82. https://doi.org/10.1007/s12546-016-9161-4

Barton, S. S., Thommasen, H. V., Tallio, B., Zhang, W., & Michalos, A. C. (2005). Health and quality of life of Aboriginal residential school survivors, Bella Coola Valley, 2001. *Social Indicators Research, 73*, 295–312. https://doi.org/10.1007/s11205-004-6169-5

Brown, S. D., Unger Hu, K. A., Mevi, A. A., Hedderson, M. M., Shan, J., Quesenberry, C. P., & Ferrara, A. (2014). The multigroup ethnic identity measure-revised: Measurement invariance across racial and ethnic groups. *Journal of Counseling Psychology, 61*(1), 154–161. https://psycnet.apa.org/doi/10.1037/a0034749

Charmaz, K. (2006). *Constructing grounded theory: A practical guide through qualitative analysis.* SAGE.

Craib, K. J., Spittal, P. M., Patel, S. H., Christian, W. M., Moniruzzaman, A., Pearce, M. E., Demerais, L., Sherlock, C. & Schechter, M. T. (2009). Prevalence and incidence of hepatitis C virus infection among Aboriginal young people who use drugs: Results from the Cedar Project. *Open Medicine, 3*(4), Article e220-7. https://europepmc.org/article/pmc/pmc3090112

Creswell, J. W. (2014). *Research design: Qualitative, quantitative, and mixed methods approaches* (4th ed.). Sage.

Distelberg, B., Williams-Reade, J., Tapanes, D., Montgomery, S., & Pandit, M. (2014). Evaluation of a family systems intervention for managing pediatric chronic illness: Mastering Each New Direction (MEND). *Family Process, 53*(2), 194–213. https://doi.org/10.1111/famp.12066

Dorion, L., & Préfontaine, D. R. (2003). *Métis land rights and self-government.* The Virtual Museum of Métis History and Culture. Gabriel Dumont Institute. https://www.metismuseum.ca/media/document.php/00725.M%C3%A9tis%20Land%20Rights.pdf

Edwards, M., & Cunningham, G. (2013). Examining the associations of perceived community racism with self-reported physical activity levels and health among older racial minority adults. *Journal of Physical Activity and Health, 10*, 932–939. https://doi.org/10.1123/jpah.10.7.932

Foulds, H. J., Shubair, M. M., & Warburton, D. E. (2013). A review of the cardiometabolic risk experience among Canadian Métis populations. *Canadian Journal of Cardiology, 29*(8), 1006–1013. https://doi.org/10.1016/j.cjca.2012.11.029

Gaudry, A. (2018). Better late than never? Canada's reluctant recognition of Métis rights and self-government. *The Indian Department* 10. Yellowhead Institute. https://yellowheadinstitute.org/2018/08/21/better-late-than-never-canadas-reluctant-recognition-of-metis-rights-and-self-government

Giroux, M. (2016). "Giving them back their spirit": Multiculturalism and resurgence at a Metis cultural festival. *MUSICultures*, 43(1), 64–88. https://journals.lib.unb.ca/index.php/MC/article/view/25260/29248

Godin, G., & Shephard, R. J. (1985). A simple method to assess exercise behavior in the community. *Canadian Journal of Applied Sport Sciences*, 10(3), 141–466.

Greenwood, M., de Leeuw, S., & Lindsay, N.M. (2018). *Determinants of Indigenous peoples' health, Second Edition: Beyond the social*. Canadian Scholars Press.

Herrington, H. M., Smith, T. B., Feinauer, E., & Griner, D. (2016). Reliability generalization of the Multigroup Ethnic Identity Measure-Revised (MEIM-R). *Journal of Counseling Psychology*, 63(5), 586–593. https://psycnet.apa.org/doi/10.1037/cou0000148

Ironside, A. K., Ferguson, L. J., Katapally, T. R., & Foulds, H. J. A. (2020). Cultural connectedness as a determinant of physical activity among Indigenous adults in Saskatchewan. *Applied Physiology, Nutrition, and Metabolism*, 45(9), 937–947. https://doi.org/10.1139/apnm-2019-0793

Ironside, A., Ferguson, L. J., Katapally, T. R., Hedayat, L. M., Johnson, S. R., & Foulds, H. J. A. (2021). Social determinants associated with physical activity among Indigenous adults at the University of Saskatchewan. *Applied Physiology, Nutrition, and Metabolism*, 46(10). https://doi.org/10.1139/apnm-2020-0781

Kahn, E. B., Ramsey, L. T., Brownson, R. C., Heath, G. W., Howze, E. H., Powell, K. E. Stone, E. J., Rajab, M. W., & Corso, P. (2002). The effectiveness of interventions to increase physical activity. A systematic review. *American Journal of Preventive Medicine*, 22(4Suppl), 73–107. https://doi.org/10.1016/S0749-3797(02)00434-8

King, M., Smith, A., & Gracey, M. (2009). Indigenous health part 2: The underlying causes of the health gap. *Lancet*, 374 (9683), 76–85. https://doi.org/10.1016/s0140-6736(09)60827-8

Kovach, M. (2009). *Indigenous methodologies: Characteristics, conversations and contexts*. University of Toronto Press.

Lavallée, L. F. (2007). Physical activity and healing through the medicine wheel. *Journal of Indigenous Wellbeing Te Mauri— Pimatisiwin*, 5(1), 127–153. https://journalindigenouswellbeing.co.nz/media/2018/10/7_Lavallee.pdf

Logan, T. (2015). Settler colonialism in Canada and the Métis. *Journal of Genocide Research*, 17(4), 433–452. https://doi.org/10.1080/14623528.2015.1096589

Macdougall, B. (2017). *Land, family and identity: Contextualizing Metis health and well-being*. National Collaborating Centre for Aboriginal Health. https://www.ccnsa-nccah.ca/docs/context/RPT-ContextualizingMetisHealth-Macdougall-EN.pdf

Mitrou, F., Cooke, M., Lawrence, D. Povah, D., Mobilia, E., Guimond, & Zubrick, S. R. (2014). Gaps in Indigenous disadvantage not closing: A census cohort study of social determinants of health in Australia, Canada, and New Zealand from 1981–2006. *BMC Public Health*, 14, Article 201. https://doi.org/10.1186/1471-2458-14-201

Monchalin, R., & Monchalin, L. (2018). Closing the health service gap: Métis women and solutions for culturally-safe health services. *Journal of Indigenous Wellbeing Te Mauri— Pimatisiwin*, 3(1), 18–29. https://journalindigenouswellbeing.co.nz/media/2022/01/109.120.Closing-the-health-service-gap-Metis-women-and-solutions-for-culturally-safe-health-services.pdf

Phinney, J. (1992). The multigroup ethnic identity measure: A new scale for use with adolescents and young adults from diverse groups. *Journal of Adolescent Research, 7*, 156–176. https://doi.org/10.1177/074355489272003

Phoenix, C. (2010). Auto-photography in aging studies: Exploring issues of identity construction in mature bodybuilders. *Journal of Aging Studies, 24*(3), 167–180. https://doi.org/10.1016/j.jaging.2008.12.007

Richardson, C. L. (2004). *Becoming Metis: The relationship between the sense of Metis self and cultural stories* [Doctoral dissertation, University of Victoria]. http://hdl.handle.net/1828/655

Richmond, C. A., Ross, N. A., & Egeland, G. M. (2007). Social support and thriving health: A new approach to understanding the health of Indigenous Canadians. *American Journal of Public Health, 97*(10), 1827–1833. https://doi.org/10.2105/AJPH.2006.096917

Roh, S., Burnette, C. E., Lee, K. H., Lee, Y. S., Easton, S. D., & M. J. Lawler. (2015). Risk and protective factors for depressive symptoms among American Indian older adults: Adverse childhood experiences and social support. *Aging & Mental Health, 19*(4), 371–380. https://doi.org/10.1080/13607863.2014.938603

Ross, R., Chaput, J. P., Giangregorio, L. M., Janssen, I., Saunders, T. J., Kho, M. E., Poitras, V. J., Tomasone, J. R., El-Kotob, R., McLaughlin, E. C., Duggan, M., Carrier, J., Carson, V., Chastin, S. F., Latimer-Cheung, A. E., Chulak-Bozzer, T., Faulkner, G., Flood, S. M., Gazendam, M. K., ... Tremblay, M. S. (2020). Canadian 24-Hour movement guidelines for adults aged 18–64 years and adults aged 65 years or older: An integration of physical activity, sedentary behaviour, and sleep. *Applied Physiology, Nutrition, and Metabolism, 45*(10, Suppl. 2), S 57–S 102. https://doi.org/10.1139/apnm-2020-0467

Sheppard, A. J., Shapiro, G. D., Bushnik, T., Wilkins, R., Perry, S., Kaufman, J. S., Kramer, M. S., & Yang, S. (2017). Birth outcomes among First Nations, Inuit and Metis populations. *Health Reports, 28*(11), 11–16. https://link.gale.com/apps/doc/A533695594/HRCA

Shore, F. (2001). The emergence of the Métis nation in Manitoba. In L. J. Barkwell, L. Dorion, and D. R. Préfontaine (Eds.), *Metis Legacy: A Metis Historiographical and Annotated Bibliography* (pp. XXX–XXX): Pemmican Publications.

Snowshoe, A., Crooks, C. V., Tremblay, P. F., Craig, W. M., & Hinson. R. E. (2015). Development of a cultural connectedness scale for First Nations youth. *Psychological Assessment, 27*(1), 249–259. https://doi.org/10.1037/a0037867

Snowshoe, A., Crooks, C. V., Tremblay, P. F., & Hinson. R. E. (2017). Cultural connectedness and its relation to mental wellness for First Nations youth. *The Journal of Primary Prevention, 38*(1–2), 67–86. https://doi.org/10.1007/s10935-016-0454-3

Walters, K. L., & Simoni, J. M. (2002). Reconceptualizing native women's health: An "indigenist" stress-coping model. *American Journal of Public Health, 92*(4), 520–524. https://doi.org/10.2105/AJPH.92.4.520

Wang, X., Liu, Q. M., Ren, Y. J., Lv, J., & Li, L. M. (2015). Family influences on physical activity and sedentary behaviours in Chinese junior high school students: A cross-sectional study. *BMC Public Health, 15*, Article 287. https://doi.org/10.1186/s12889-015-1593-9

Williams, D. R. (1999). Race, socioeconomic status, and health: The added effects of racism and discrimination. *Annals of the New York Academy of Science*, 896, 173–188. https://doi.org/10.1111/j.1749-6632.1999.tb08114.x

Wilson, D., & Macdonald, D. (2010). The income gap between Aboriginal peoples and the rest of Canada. Canadian Centre for Policy Alternatives. https://policyalternatives.ca/sites/default/files/uploads/publications/reports/docs/Aboriginal%20Income%20Gap.pdf

· 9 ·

THE GRANDMOTHERS OF THE PRAIRIES TO WOODLANDS INDIGENOUS LANGUAGE REVITALIZATION CIRCLE

Laura Forsythe

> Along with our partner organizations, we are honored to be working to revive and revitalize Michif and other Métis and Indigenous languages, while connecting communities across borders, boundaries and generations.
>
> — Verna DeMontigny and Heather Souter

Daañ lii Michif leu teeraeñ d'niikinaahk eekwaa Daañ lii Anishinaabeg, lii Krii, lii Oji-Krii, lii Syoo pi lii Dene nishtam leu peeyii, lii kampoos d'yuniversitii di Manitoba ashteewa.[1] The University of Winnipeg campuses are located on the original lands of Anishinaabeg, Cree, Oji-Cree, Dakota, and Dene peoples, and the homeland of the Métis nation; this is where I live, work, and study. I also want to acknowledge that the power provided to write this chapter was created in Treaty 5 territory and that the water in my tea came from Shoal Lake. Following the model of Métis scholars like LaRocque (1975, 2015a), Acoose (1995), and Adese et al. (2017), a Métis introduction begins the chapter to describe the researcher and contextualize the conversation: Laura Forsythe d-ishinikaashon more fully. My name is Laura Forsythe. Ma famii kawyesh Roostertown d-oshciwak. My family was from Rooster Town a long time ago. Anosh ma famii Winnipeg wikiwak. Today my family lives in Winnipeg. Ma Parentii (my ancestors) are Huppe, Ward, Berard,

Morin, Lavallee, and Cyr. The three grandmothers featured in this chapter have begun to teach me Southern Michif, one of my ancestors' languages.

This chapter celebrates the contributions of three Michif grandmothers—Grace Zoldy, Verna DeMontigny, and Heather Souter—to the Prairies to Woodlands Indigenous Language Revitalization Circle (P2WILRC) and thus to the revitalization of Michif through community work taken into the academy. P2WILRC is a grassroots non-profit established in 2018 and focused on revitalizing Southern Michif and other Indigenous languages spoken by the Métis and our kin. The circle's efforts have included a variety of approaches, such as a master–apprentice program, immersion camps, and social media groups to build community, along with online resources.

In partnership with SoundHunters, P2WILRC participated in a research project exploring the efficacy of language learning by repurposing a digital gaming system (Lothian, 2022). In 2022, P2WILRC launched Michif.org, a website that houses three critical resources. The first involves working with 7000 languages to create a free 20-unit, 61-lesson online course: *Southern Michif Course Aapachihtaataak li "Online Course"!* (Transparent Language, 2021). Second, the *Michif Mother Tongue Dictionary* (Mother Tongues, 2021) digitized Laverdure and Allard's (1983) *Turtle Mountain Michif Dictionary*, adapting it to the Southern Michif context by providing audio for over 15,384 words in the voices of Verna DeMontigny, Connie Henry, Heather Souter, and Grace Zoldy. Third, Michif.org includes a verb conjugator that creates well-formed verbs in Michif for learners seeking to build sentences.

The grandmothers that founded P2WILRC began their journeys in Southern Michif language revitalization long before coming together in the late 2010s. This chapter explores and highlights their decades of work prior to the successes of the non-profit in recent years. This relation of past work, as Welsh (1991) notes, is "affirmation of the importance of women's experience; affirmation of strength, courage, resilience of our grandmothers; affirmation of our ability to speak both of our past and our present to make our voices heard" (p. 24). Holding these women up as grandmothers aligns with Campbell's thoughts (2007) on the role of grandmothers as our first teachers. According to Iseke and Desmoulins (2011), grandmothers "reflect Métis sensibilities and move beyond the roles of child rearing and carrying families" (p. 24). This quote speaks to the reality that the women in this chapter do not all have children but have all conceived of ways of thinking about the Michif. The words shared by these three Métis women to save Michif confirm Iseke and Desmoulins's (2011) view that grandmothers share narratives as community historians, expressing the confidence and pride of our people and vital to those who walk behind. Flaminio et al. (2020), Forsythe (2022), and Hodgson-Smith and Kermoal (2016) speak to the role of grandmothers in *wahkootowin* in transmitting the knowledge embedded in the actions of these three women.

This chronicle of their contributions reveals themes in their publications, which include nation-sponsored publications, academic citations, non-Indigenous scholars' use of these publications to build their careers, using the grandmothers' work in doctoral research, and their tenacity in saving Southern Michif from extinction.

Most of their early work was sponsored by the Métis nation or its affiliated research institutions like the Gabriel Dumont Institute, the Louis Riel Institute, or the Métis-owned Pemmican Publications. This reality may speak to a bias against historians without Western educations documenting the past in the academy or the support given to Métis scholarship before the 1990s by the Manitoba Métis Federation (MMF). Notably, the scholars who cite these women, outside of Maria Campbell, are primarily not Métis. This theme speaks to the grandmothers' work being unknown due to being released by obscure publishers or sponsored by the nation; these women were ignored in the academy for generations unless non-Métis scholars cited them. The increase in citations of many of these grandmothers starting in the present century indicates an increase in their profiles: they are all award-winning and cited hundreds of times and yet are scarcely present in many Métis scholars' work. This exclusion speaks to the need to raise their profiles within the Métis community and establish their existence outside of external sources.

The second theme that emerges from these grandmothers' contributions is the sheer volume of their publications' uptake into academia, as they are cited in numerous publications to argue or shore up scholarly work and build careers off the backs of Métis women. Despite these works primarily originating in mainstream publishing houses or Métis-sponsored ones, their work is used throughout academia. The timeframe of the publications (starting in the 1980s) and the scarcity of Métis scholars conducting academic publishing resulted in numerous non-Métis or non-First Nations scholars using these early publications. However, in some cases following the 1990s, non-Indigenous scholars consistently did not possess any knowledge. Linguists such as Nicole Rosen, Peter Bakker, Olivia Sammons, and Maria Mazzoli, even after decades of publications in Michif, continue to rely on these grandmothers as they have yet to acquire the language in which they are experts.

Another theme detailed below is the inclusion of these grandmothers in doctoral research. Unsurprisingly, citations of these grandmothers' work, beginning in the 1980s and continuing through the present day, can be found in dissertations.

Grace Zoldy (Ledoux)

Born in 1933 in Camperville, Manitoba, to a family of fluent Michif speakers, Zoldy has been acknowledged in many highly influential publications on Michif. The 2010 Ka Ni Kanichihk Keeping the Fires Burning Award recipient stated, "This is not for me. This is for my people" (Martin & Bonneville, 2010) when speaking of all the work done to revitalize Michif.

Zoldy's academic contributions to our current grasp of Michif are profound when broken down into three groups: understanding modality, participating in documentation, and teaching the language. Bakker (1997) highlights Zoldy's contributions to all three in a critically acclaimed book on the genesis of Michif. Rosenblum and Sammons (2014) feature the work of Zoldy in documenting the multimodal nature of the language, while Gillon and Rosen praise her for her work on "Critical Mass in Michif" (2016), as she provided all the article's original fieldwork and data. More recently, Gillon et al. (2018) featured Zoldy's contributions to the language in depicting the evolution of Michif over time, and Cox and Sammons (2019) acknowledge Zoldy for documenting language variation. In terms of teaching Michif, Sammons (2013), Barkwell, Dorian, and Carrière-Acco (2009, 2012, 2019), and Adam (2020) all include Zoldy's work in this area, highlighting the master–apprentice language learning program aimed at creating new fluent Michif speakers. Zoldy contributed to publications such as *Piikishkweetak aa'n Michif* (Rosen & Souter, 2009b), a textbook that supports adult Michif language courses, and was the sole editor of *Li liiv oche Michif ayamiiawina: The Book of Michif Prayers* (2009), which documents 16 prayers in both Michif and English. These prayers had previously been featured in *Metis Legacy II* (Barkwell, Dorion, & Hourie, 2006), to which Zoldy contributed; Mazzoli (2020) captures her contributions to language revitalization while acknowledging the challenges that remain.

Zoldy's efforts to teach Michif and understand its linguistics are featured in the work of several graduate students, such as Rosen (2007), who cites Zoldy alongside Norman Fleury and Rita Flamand: "I would be nowhere without these three people, and I am so glad they agree to share their knowledge with me" (p. v). Likewise, McCreery (2013) writes, "I want to acknowledge my Michif teacher, Grace Zoldy, for giving me my language, without which I would not have been able to do this research" (p. vii). Both scholars have since become prolific in linguistics and language revitalization.

Zoldy's contributions go beyond the language of Michif, with Edge and McCallum (2006) documenting her stories at a Métis Elders gathering and Castellano et al. (2008) recording Zoldy's recollections of her time in Christ the King School in Camperville as part of their documentation of the Métis experience at residential schools.

Verna DeMontigny

Verna DeMontigny was born in 1951 in Li Kwayn (the Corner), 7½ miles from Binscarth, Manitoba. However, her parents were from a community called Ste. Madeline on the Saskatchewan–Manitoba border, and her family names are Fleury, Ledoux, Gendron, LaPointe, and DeMontigny. She is a champion of Michif and has dedicated much of her life to its preservation; in 2003, she was named an Elder of the National Task Force on Aboriginal Languages and Cultures (Barkwell, 2018). As with so many Métis grandmothers, DeMontigny's work in the community is undocumented; however, Barkwell (2018) speaks to her decades of work teaching and documenting Michif, including at the University of Winnipeg, the University of Manitoba, and Brandon University. For 15 years, DeMontigny worked with Aboriginal Head Start programs and K–12 schools in Brandon to save a critically endangered language. Then, in 2010, DeMontigny spent five years coordinating the Michif Language Program in the MMF Southwest Region, serving Portage la Prairie, Minnedosa, Brandon, Turtle Mountain (Boissevain), Binscarth, and St. Ambroise.

DeMontigny has participated in several initiatives geared toward saving Michif over the years, including serving as a board member of the P2WILRC, which uses the master–apprentice Indigenous language revitalization model to create fluent speakers of five Indigenous languages (DeMontigny, 2019b). In addition, DeMontigny has been crucial to the inclusion of Michif on the National Center for Collaboration in Indigenous Education resource website, with *Aakoota-kaawaapaamittin: The Michif Language* (DeMontigny, 2019a) and sat for a recording during a Michif gathering at the University of Manitoba (DeMontigny, 2019b).

DeMontigny recently co-authored several linguistic articles surrounding Michif's nominal contact, phonology, and syntax; for example, Gillon et al. (2018) document language contact using DeMontigny's role as the central knowledge keeper of the Michif language. She is cited in works such as Sammons's doctoral dissertation (2019) and papers by Rosen et al. (2019, 2020), Mazzoli (2020, 2021), and O'Shannessy (2020). In addition, Michif is featured in *The Routledge Handbook of Language Contact* (2020). Its inclusion in that handbook speaks to the significant impact that Métis women who are fluent Michif speakers—like Anne Anderson-Irvine, Rita Flamand, Grace Zoldy, and DeMontigny herself—have had in academia; their ability to help create successful careers for non-Indigenous and non-Michif-speaking linguists is documented through the publications above, as none of those authors speaks Michif.

Rosenblum and Sammons (2014), Rosen and Souter (2015), Sammons (2015), Cox and Sammons (2019), Rosen et al. (2019), and Mattes (2021) all acknowledge DeMontigny as a transcriptionist and translator for their work; each has an academic following that is now taking up her knowledge. *Piikishkweetak aa'n Michif!* (Rosen & Souter, 2009b) is a teacher's manual for Michif teachers that relies on DeMontigny's ability to speak Michif. Interestingly, Bakker (1997) and Bakker and Papen (1997) acknowledge many speakers but exclude DeMontigny, despite her being a fluent Michif speaker. However, decades later, Mazzoli, Bakker, and DeMontigny worked together on a book chapter (2021).

DeMontigny also champions the remembrance of her home community, Ste. Madeleine, which the Government of Manitoba stole to provide pastures for farmers (Manitoba Museum, 2019). To preserve this history, the "Ni KishKishin, I Remember Ste. Madeleine's" exhibition was translated into Michif by DeMontigny, whose parents were survivors of the razing in 1938. Sammons (2013) features DeMontigny's translations in *Leaving Ste. Madeleine: A Michif Account* articulates the experience of the 200 people affected by the government's decision to prioritize cattle over the Métis community.

Although now retired as a teacher, DeMontigny's contributions to academia appear to be only beginning. She is involved in a number of projects under review with University of Manitoba Press in collaboration with the P2WILRC, such as a new audio-video documentation project focusing on the activities and language functions of everyday life and Michif and Métis culture as lived by their family, ongoing master–apprentice work, Michif language videos for learners, Michif dictionary recordings, online Michif workshops, a translation of an Ojibwe book for language learners into Michif, oral translations of Michif radio recordings from 1985 to 1995 (from radio station KEYA in Belcourt, North Dakota), and beta-testing a verb conjugator, all while making guest appearances in Michif language classes at the University of Manitoba (Heather Souter, personal communication, August 16, 2021).

In 2023, DeMontigny was awarded the Order of Gabriel Dumont by the Gabriel Dumont Institute for her service to the Métis of Canada with distinction. DeMontigny's contributions to the revitalization of Michif demonstrate the strength and knowledge Métis women can bring to Métis scholarship and the Métis nation.

Heather Souter

Souter, a language activist working to revitalize Michif, was born in Vancouver, British Columbia, in 1962. Her Métis kinship ties stem from Fish Creek, Fort di Plains, Slave Lake, and Lac St. Anne, Alberta, including her great-grandmother Julie Marie Belcourt. Souter married into the Camperville community decades ago and is now an MMF citizen working alongside the organization to revitalize Michif. Her family names are Belcourt, Campion, Sapin/Sapendit, L'Hirondelle, and Nipissing. Souter insists that she carries out this work from a grassroots perspective. However, her academic contributions to our grasp of Michif are profound when broken down into four groups: understanding the linguistics of Michif, documenting the language, mentoring, and teaching Michif.

Souter credits her language revitalization and linguistics expertise to years of working with Métis matriarchs Grace Zoldy and Rita Flamand in both the community and the academy, culminating in her master's thesis (2018b). Since graduating, Souter has co-authored several articles. For example, Brinklow et al. (2019) describe the historical and social context of Indigenous language technology in Canada and note the benefit of having the community work further to save languages. Kuhn et al. (2020) survey a project that assists Indigenous communities in Canada in developing software for language revitalization. Davis et al. (2021) focus on the computational modeling of Michif verbal morphology in a paper that presents a finite-state computational model of the verbal morphology of Michif. Finally, Mazzoli (2021) uses unpublished material and cites it as Souter (2010), including an index of verb finals for Michif to increase our understanding of the morphology of Michif.

Rosen and Souter's *Piikishkweetak aa'n Michif* (2009b) is a teaching aid that affirms Michif spelling conventions and provides documentation of

Michif possessives in French and hybrid systems. It served as a basis for several linguistic modeling efforts by Sammons (2013, 2019) and Mazzoli (2019, 2020, 2021). In addition, Rosen and Souter (2015) use the Flamand-Papen spelling system created by Rita Flamand and Robert Papen and provide affirmation for the way forward in conventional spelling for Michif.

Souter (2007) asserts the need to document the Michif language's status as severely endangered and informs readers that most first-language speakers are over 70 years old, making immediate data collection urgent. Souter has presented worldwide on the subject, and Rosen and Souter's (2009a, 2009b) work is widely cited because it speaks to multilingual communities like those in Ste. Madeleine (Sammons, 2013).

One of the roles that grandmothers and aunties of Métis scholarship have played in the academy is mentoring emerging—and established—scholars, a principle of *wahkootowin*. Souter is acknowledged in Rosen's (2007) work documenting the phonology of Michif: "Heather Souter has pushed me to learn more about the Michif people and language and has been a source of inspiration, as she lives and learns the Michif language" (p. v). Fowler (2022) and Ferland (2022) describe Souter's teachings as an aid to their understanding of Métisness and Michif. Huang's (2010) work discussing language revitalization and identity politics also thanks Souter for guidance. Mazzoli (2019, 2020) explores the challenges and celebrations in the revitalization of Michif in two papers that thank Souter for consultation. Finally, Sammons (2019), whose doctoral work outlines nominal classification in Michif, cites Souter heavily, including thanking her "for introducing and encouraging me to work on Michif" (p. vii).

Souter has provided translations for numerous mainstream publications. Newland (2022) and O'Brien (2015) cite Souter's work with children's author Julia Flett in *Owls See Clearly at Night (Lii Yiiboo Nayaapiwak lii Swer): A Michif Alphabet*. Souter (2004) reviews a model for language revitalization that is the basis of the master-apprenticeship program facilitated by the P2WILRC, the non-profit co-founded by Souter and Verna DeMontigny. The National Center for Indigenous Education published a video featuring Souter discussing the model (Souter, 2019).

Committed to more than the pursuit of academic achievement, Souter developed video resources to support independent adult language learning (2018a). Coming after other Michif language teaching tools, such as Rosen and Souter (2009b, 2015), the Michif textbook includes a 12-week self-guided lesson plan heralded by the Métis nation and scholars as an essential part of revitalizing Michif. Souter also created the Michif Verb Rummy game (2008) to encourage learners to spend recreational time with the language.

As an educator, Souter has taught in community and post-secondary settings for over a decade. In 2018 she advocated for the inclusion of Michif I and II in the Department of Indigenous Studies at the University of Manitoba (Forsythe, 2022). Since the course's inception, Souter has provided over 325 learners with an introduction to Michif. In 2022, the University of Winnipeg hired Souter as an assistant professor in the Department of Anthropology.

Conclusion

In conclusion, this chapter sought to bring to our collective attention the actions and contributions made by the founders of P2WILRC—Grace Zoldy, Verna DeMontigny, and Heather Souter—over the past five decades in an effort to reclaim and revitalize Southern Michif. Through a chronicle of their contributions, three themes emerged regarding Métis grandmothers' contributions to the academy and language revitalization. Their work should be remembered, as our language will live on because of their tenacity and dedication to the Métis people.

Note

1 This is written in Southern Michif.

References

Adam, B. A. (2020, September/October). Kahkiihtwaam ee-pee-kiiweetataahk: Bringing it back home again. *Canadian Geographic, 140*, 32–45. https://www.canadiangeographic.ca/article/kahkiihtwaam-ee-pee-kiiweehtataahk-bringing-it-back-home-again

Bakker, P. (1997). *A language of our own: The genesis of Michif, the mixed Cree-French language of the Canadian Métis*. Oxford University Press.

Bakker, P., & Papen, R. A. (1997). Michif: A mixed language based on Cree and French. In S. G. Thomason (Ed.), *Contact languages: A wider perspective* (pp. 295–363). John Benjamins. https://doi.org/10.1075/cll.17.12bak

Barkwell, L. J. (2018). *Verna DeMontigny née Fleury*. The Virtual Museum of Métis History and Culture. http://www.metismuseum.ca/media/document.php/149499.Verna%20DeMontigny%20n%C3%A9e%20Fleury.pdf

Barkwell, L. J., Dorion, L., & Hourie, A. (2006). *Metis legacy II: Michif culture, heritage, and folkways*. Gabriel Dumont Institute.

Barkwell, L. J., Dorion, L., & Carrière-Acco, A. (2009). *Women of the Métis Nation*. Gabriel Dumont Institute Press.

Barkwell, L. J., Dorion, L., & Carrière-Acco, A. (2012). *Women of the Métis Nation* (2nd ed.). Gabriel Dumont Institute Press.

Barkwell, L. J., Dorion, L., & Carrière-Acco, A. (2019). *Women of the Métis Nation* (3rd ed.). Gabriel Dumont Institute Press.

Barkwell, L. J., Dorion, L., Hourie, A., & Zoldy, G. (2009). *Métis death rituals and ceremonies*. The Virtual Museum of Métis History and Culture. Gabriel Dumont Institute. http://www.metismuseum.ca/media/document.php/11728.Metis%20Death%20Ceremonies.pdf

Brinklow, N. T., Littell, P., Lothian, D., Pine, A., & Souter, H. (2019). Indigenous language technologies & language reclamation in Canada. In G. Adda, K. Choukri, I. Kasinskaite-Buddeberg, J. Mariani, H. Mazo, & S. Saktriani (Eds.), *Collection of research papers of the 1st International Conference on Language Technologies for All* (pp. 402–406). https://lt4all.elra.info/proceedings/lt4all2019/pdf/2019.lt4all-1.100.pdf

Canadian Heritage. (2021). *A week focused on Indigenous-led efforts to reclaim, revitalize, maintain and strengthen Indigenous languages: Highlights of new projects funded in Western Canada*. https://www.newswire.ca/news-releases/a-week-focused-on-indigenous-led-efforts-to-reclaim-revitalize-maintain-and-strengthen-indigenous-languages-highlights-of-new-projects-funded-in-western-canada-841593135.html

Castellano, M. B., Davis, L., & Lahache, L. (Eds.). (2000). *Aboriginal education: Fulfilling the promise*. UBC Press.

Chew, K. A., Child, S., Sammons, O., & Souter, H. (2022). *Learning in relation – Creating Online Indigenous language courses: Benefits to the community (Part 3/4)*. University of Victoria. http://hdl.handle.net/1828/14548

Cox, C., & Sammons, O. N. (2019). *Bridging the gap: Incorporating language variation into documentary and descriptive linguistics* [PowerPoint slides]. LD&C. https://scholarspace.manoa.hawaii.edu/server/api/core/bitstreams/4e72a146-56d7-4cb2-8768-999bb8094ad0/content

Davis, F., Santos, E. A., & Souter, H. (2021). On the computational modelling of Michif verbal morphology. In *Proceedings of the 16th Conference of the European Chapter of the Association for Computational Linguistics* (pp. 2631–2636). Association for Computational Linguistics. https://aclanthology.org/2021.eacl-main.226.pdf

DeMontigny, V. (2019a). *Aakoota-kaawaapaamittin: The Michif language* [Video]. National Center for Collaboration in Indigenous Education. https://www.nccie.ca/story/aakoota-kaawaapaamittin-the-michif-language/

DeMontigny, V. (2019b). *Michif language gathering: Verna DeMontigny* [Video]. National Center for Collaboration in Indigenous Education. https://www.youtube.com/watch?v=bb8C3WH3Fk8&t=1s

Edge, L., & McCallum, T. (2006). Métis identity: Sharing traditional knowledge and healing practices at Métis elders' gatherings. *Pimatisiwin: A Journal of Aboriginal & Indigenous Community Health*, 4(2), 83–115. http://www.pimatisiwin.com/uploads/1399918655.pdf

Gillon, C., & Rosen, N. (2016). Critical mass in Michif. *Journal of Pidgin and Creole Languages*, *31*(1), 113–140. https://doi.org/10.1075/jpcl.31.1.05gil

Gillon, C., & Rosen, N., with DeMontigny, V. (2018). *Nominal contact in Michif*. Oxford University Press.

Ferland, N. A. (2022). *"We're still here": Teaching and learning about Métis women's and two-spirit people's relationships with land in Winnipeg* [Master's Thesis, University of Saskatchewan]. https://hdl.handle.net/10388/13931

Forsythe, L. (2022). Easing the culture shock of being in a space dominated by the educated. *Aboriginal Policy studies*, *10*(1). https://doi.org/10.5663/aps.v10i1.29405.

Fowler, L. (2022). *Where learning happens: Conversations with queer, Métis youth who engage in hip-hop cultures* [Doctoral dissertation, University of Saskatchewan]. https://hdl.handle.net/10388/13941

Huang, C. J. (2010). *Language revitalization and identity politics: An examination of Siraya reclamation in Taiwan*. [Doctoral dissertation, University of Florida]. http://hdl.handle.net/10125/5013

Kuhn, R., Davis, F., Désilets, A., Joanis, E., Kazantseva, A., Knowles, R., Littell, P. Lothian, D., Pine, A., Running Wolf, C., Santos, E., Stewart, D., Boulianne, G., Gupta, V., Owennatékha, B. M., Martin, A., Cox, C. Junker, M.-O., Sammons, O., ... Souter, H. (2020). The Indigenous Languages Technology project at NRC Canada: An empowerment-oriented approach to developing language software. In D. Scott, N. Bel, & C. Zong (Eds.), *Proceedings of the 28th International Conference on Computational Linguistics* (pp. 5866–5878). Association for Computational Linguistics. http://dx.doi.org/10.18653/v1/2020.coling-main.516

Laverdure, P., & Allard, I. R. (1983). *The Michif dictionary: Turtle Mountain Chippewa Cree*. Pemmican Publications.

Lothian, D. (2022). *Southern Michif SoundHunters: A collaborative process of re-purposing an Indigenous language learning technology* [Master's thesis, University of Alberta].

Manitoba Museum. (2019, May 24). *Métis story finally being told, in Michif, at the Manitoba Museum*. https://manitobamuseum.ca/metis-story-finally-being-told-in-michif-at-the-manitoba-museum/

Martin, M., & Bonneville, R. (2010, September 25) La lang di Michif ta-pashipiikan: That means, "The Michif language will survive." Perhaps it's true. *Winnipeg Free Press*. https://www.winnipegfreepress.com/local/la-lang-di-michif-ta-pashipiikan-103776389.html

Mattes, C. (2021). *Indigenous littoral curation: A viable framework for collaborative and dialogic curatorial practice* [Doctoral dissertation, University of Manitoba]. https://mspace.lib.umanitoba.ca/handle/1993/35440

Mazzoli, M. (2019). Michif loss and resistance in four Métis communities: Kahkiyaw mashchineenaan, "All of us are disappearing as in a plague." *Zeitschrift für Kanada-Studien*, *39*, 96–117. http://www.kanada-studien.org/wp-content/uploads/2021/02/zks_2019_5_Mazzoli.pdf

Mazzoli, M. (2020). Michif studies: Challenges and opportunities in collaborative language research. *Journal of Postcolonial Linguistics*, *3*, 43–63. https://iacpl.net/wp-content/uploads/2020/06/Mazzoli.pdf

Mazzoli, M. (2021). Secondary derivation in the Michif verb: Beyond the traditional Algonquian template. In D. M. Perez & E. Sippola (Eds.), *Postcolonial language varieties in the Americas* (pp. 81–180). De Gruyter. https://doi.org/10.1515/9783110723977-005

Mazzoli, M., Bakker, P., & DeMontigny, V. (2021). Michif mixed verbs: Typologically unusual word-internal mixing. In M. Mazzoli & E. Sippola (Eds.), *New perspectives on mixed languages: From core to fringe* (pp. 121–156). De Gruyter Mouton.

McCreery, D. (2013). *Challenges and solutions in adult acquisition of Cree as a second language* [Master's thesis, University of Victoria]. https://dspace.library.uvic.ca/bitstream/handle/1828/4584/McCreery_Dale_MA_2013.pdf?sequence=5&isAllowed=y

Newland, J. (2022). Seeing through the dark, breaking through the silence: An interview with Julie Flett. *Jeunesse: Young People, Texts, Cultures, 14*(1), 84–103. https://doi.org/10.3138/jeunesse-14.1.06

O'Brien, S. (2015). Meet Julie Flett: Book Week Artist: The award winning Cree-Métis artist, Julie Flett, talks to the Canadian Children's Book Centre's Sandra O'Brien about her work, her recent books and her First Nation Communities READ tour. *Canadian Children's Book News, 38*(1), 18–20.

O'Shannessy, C. (2020). Mixed languages. In In E. Adamou & Y. Matras (Eds.), *The Routledge handbook of language contact* (pp. 325–348). Routledge.

Rosen, N. (2007). *Domains in Michif phonology* [Doctoral dissertation, University of Toronto].

Rosen, N. & Souter, H. (2009a, March 12–14). *Language revitalization in a multilingual community: The case of Michif* [Paper presentation]. 1st Annual International Conference on Language Documentation and Conservation, Honolulu, HI, United States. http://hdl.handle.net/10125/5090.

Rosen, N., & Souter, H. (2009b). *Piikishkweetak aa'n Michif!* Louis Riel Institute.

Rosen, N., & Souter, H. (2015). *Piikishkweetak aa'n Michif!* (2nd ed.). Manitoba Métis Federation.

Rosen, N., Stewart, J., Pesch-Johnson, M., & Sammons, O. N. (2019). *Michif VOT.* http://www.jessestewart.net/uploads/1/8/8/0/18807788/rosen_nicole_jesse_stewart_michele_pesch-johnson_olivia_sammons--2019--vot_in_michif.pdf

Rosen, N., Stewart, J., & Sammons, O. N. (2020). How "mixed" is mixed language phonology? An acoustic analysis of the Michif vowel system. *The Journal of the Acoustical Society of America, 147*(4), 2989–2999. https://doi.org/10.1121/10.0001009

Rosenblum, D., & Sammons, O. N. (2014, January 2–5). *Documenting multimodal interaction: Workflows, data management, and archiving* [PowerPoint presentation]. Linguistic Society of America 2014 Annual Meeting, Minneapolis, MN, United States. https://www.linguisticsociety.org/sites/default/files/Rosenblum_Sammons-Documenting_Multimodal_Interaction.pdf

Sammons, O. N. (2013). Leaving Ste. Madeleine: A Michif account. *The Canadian Journal of Native Studies, 33*(2), 149–164.

Sammons, O. (2015, March 12). *From technical to teachable: The role of texts in documentation and pedagogy* [Paper presentation]. 4th International Conference on Language Documentation and Conversation (ICLDC), Honolulu, HI, United States. http://hdl.handle.net/10125/25374

Sammons, O. (2019). *Nominal classification in Michif* [Doctoral dissertation, University of Alberta]. https://doi.org/10.7939/r3-b8sq-xz05

Souter, H. M. (2004). [Review of *How to keep your language alive: A common sense approach to one-on-one language learning*, by L. Hinton (with M. Vera & N. Steele)]. *International Journal of American Linguistics*, 70(4), 456–458. https://doi.org/10.1086/429210

Souter, H. (2007). Michif, the "mixed language" of the Métis: The need for documentation. *KU Anthropologist*, 19(2–3).

Souter, H. (2008). Michif verb rummy. http://www.Metismuseum.ca/browse/index.php/987

Souter, H. (2010). An index of verb finals in Michif. An inventory of abstract and complex verb finals using the Michif dictionary Turtle Mountain Chippewa Cree as corpus. University of Lethbridge [Term project for Ling 5990: Michif Morphology].

Souter, H. (2018a, July 26). A guide to *Ti Parii Chiiñ*: Michif master-apprentice survival phrases and micro grammar lessons [Video]. https://www.youtube.com/watch?v=-qwd1QjcLi-Y&t=0s&list=PLI2E8ojtLxiZnsi1-V67w_NJcoJDLGS7c&index=2

Souter, H. (2018b). Ti parii chiiñ? (Are you ready?): Preparing adult learners and proficient speakers for the challenge of Michif reclamation [Unpublished Master's thesis, University of Victoria].

Souter, H. (2019). *Master-apprentice Indigenous language revitalization in Michif and other Indigenous languages* [Video]. The National Center for Indigenous Education. https://www.nccie.ca/story/master-apprentice-Indigenous-language-revitalization-in-michif-and-other-Indigenous-languages/

Transparent Language. (2021). *Southern Michif Course Aapachihtaataak li "Online Course"!* https://michif.org/online-course/

Zoldy, G. L. (2009). *Li liivr oche Michif ayamiiawina–The book of Michif prayers*. Pemmican.

· 10 ·

LI KEUR, RIEL'S HEART OF THE NORTH, AN ARTISTIC NARRATION OF MÉTIS HISTORY THROUGH PEOPLEHOOD: ADDRESSING MÉTIS (MIS)RECOGNITION AND RECENTERING MÉTIS WOMEN

Suzanne M. Steele, with an introduction by Nicole Stonyk

Operatic and other works portraying Louis Riel are not new to Canada's classical music scene. Over the last 50 years, Riel has been used in a variety of genres, including choral works, musicals, and full-scale operas. The narratives of Louis Riel in musical contexts often center on his trial and hanging and participate in the mythmaking enterprise of Riel as madman, martyr, and religious prophet. A welcome departure from Eurocentric and masculinist depictions of Riel and Métis people appears in a dramatic musical work called Li Keur: Riel's Heart of the North. This musical work was selected as a historic re-investment in the arts to showcase diversity and artistic expressions in celebration of the 150th anniversary of Confederation and challenges the classical music hierarchy and the Eurocentric aesthetic that is common in contemporary Indigenous performance works. The following chapter is written by Suzanne Steele, librettist and Indigenous lead for Li Keur: Riel Heart of the North. Most importantly, the words of Steele are used in this platform as a Métis woman and librettist and storyteller to push against the paternalistic and ageist hierarchies commonly associated within the classical music sector. Steele's words live here to represent her experiences and intentions as a librettist and the artistic process that is often diminished in general narratives surrounding musical performances. Li Keur transcends, changes, and reinterprets the historical narrative established by previous musical iterations of Louis Riel through "who" tells "our" history and when relationships and value systems are recentered.

Over the past 150-plus years, there have been numerous plays, musicals, poems and poetry collections, reports, a graphic novel, a three-hour CBC television broadcast, and many other retellings of Métis leader Louis Riel's life (1844–1885). Most of these have centered on his politics, his trial, and his execution—many with a particular focus on his personal travails and/or his "madness."[1] In 1979, the Canadian Broadcasting Corporation produced a three-part dramatization, *Riel*, written by Roy Moore, "an Eastern Canadian non-Metis playwright" (Walz et al., 1981). In one of three reviews of the series published by the Manitoba Historical Society, Métis historian Emma Larocque observes that "the most disturbing aspect of the film is that while it magnifies Riel, it almost entirely neglects the Metis community" (Walz et al., 1981).[2] Clearly, mainstream producers of English Canadian culture failed Riel and the Métis people in 1979 in much in the same way as the Harry Somers and Mavor Moore opera *Louis Riel* had failed a decade earlier. Arguably, so too did the 2017 remount of the Riel opera by the Canadian Opera Company (COC), about which I write about in greater detail below.[3] Despite all this failure and clearly throwing caution to the wind (yes, a cliché, but opera is full of delicious clichés) and fully knowing that there will be critics of my work no matter what I write, I wrote the book and libretti, and envisioned a new opera on Riel. This opera, *Li Keur* ("the heart" in Michif), *Riel's Heart of the North*, with composers Neil Weisensel (newcomer) and Alex Kusturok (Métis), previewed in 2019 with the RSO and a stellar, predominantly Indigenous cast and is scheduled to be produced in full in 2023.[4]

That I would attempt to write another major piece on Riel raised a question: "Am I also mad?"[5] In this chapter, I provide the context of why I wrote about Riel and my approach to a story that could easily have had a hundred operas written about it, as with any aspect of Riel's life. I also look at the Métisness of my methodologies, or as I prefer to say, my approaches, in the creation of the opera. In this I wonder if it is possible that an inherent Métisness exists in this artistic practice, as I believe in my work one can locate a cultural longing, a distinct notion to transcend expectations, despite years of formal training as a classical singer and a musician with a music degree. And I contemplate the challenges of my approaches—how I envision the work, and how I write and then refine the work. I also discuss the many personal and artistic challenges I have experienced along the way. But first, I provide the context of the project.

In 2017, after being introduced to the composer Neil Weisensel by our mutual agent, Ian Arnold, we determined the time might be right to create a new opera on Louis Riel. This was the same year that the COC remounted the opera *Louis Riel* by Harry Somers (composer) and Mavor Moore (librettist). The 1967 opera, originally commissioned for Canada's centenary, was at the time considered revolutionary in that the subject was the controversial Indigenous leader. But to remount it was problematic, partly for its modernist musical language, as Robert Harris notes in his 2017 review; it has the "quasi-dissonant, highly angular, international style in the mid-sixties"; it is, frankly, unpalatable to lay people's ears. But the more fundamental reason that many Métis people feel it should not have been remounted is that the work was not created by anyone within the Métis community, even as a collaborator.

With the provenance of Riel productions in mind and believing that it was time for a Métis-driven collaboration, I took the leap with Weisensel; we applied for and received one of the large Canada 150 Canada Council New Chapter awards to create *Li Keur*. But when I describe it as an opera, I wonder if *Li Keur* can really be described as such. Certainly, Weisensel (a newcomer and co-director of the project)[6] and I have debated this for most of the five years we have worked on it; at times we consider it an opera, at other times a dramatic musical, and sometimes, as when it encompassed a SSHRC-sponsored, Indigenous language research project, it has been a musical, cultural, and linguistic collaboration couched within a paradigm of reconciliation (Steele, n.d.).[7] Yet to frame *Li Keur* as a project of reconciliation understates the enormity of that task; instead, it might be looked at as a small step in the direction of reconciliation (with many steps backward); Indigenous Elders have told us we are "doing it right" as we work carefully with many communities, adhering to protocols, working with their timelines, and forming relationships.[8]

The story, the libretti, and the book of *Li Keur* are wholly conceived by me, with the text set to music by composers Neil Weisensel and Alex Kusturok, a Métis fiddler. Kusturok, a North American fiddle champion (with lightning footwork) was brought in during the process of composition because I believed his Métis voice was needed, just as translators were needed in the composition of my original text: they Indigenized rather than exoticized.

Li Keur, then, rather than being described as an opera might best be described as the result of large theatrical gathering that consist of many visits with symphony orchestra players, conductors, fiddlers, jiggers, classically trained soloists, adult and children's Métis choruses, actor–narrators, and many, many community members (Indigenous and newcomer). In 2018, *Li Keur* was workshopped in Winnipeg with Indigenous and newcomer singers, the Métis fiddler Melissa Goddard, and pianist Cary Denby. In 2019, 45 minutes of *Li Keur* previewed in Regina with the Regina Symphony Orchestra (RSO).[9] These performances were extremely well received by audience members, but what was significant for me was the reaction of the choruses, who told me how moved they were to be hearing and singing in Michif and Anishinaabemowin; some of them were hearing their own languages for the first time in their lives.

Structurally, it is challenging to peg this work, a piece that is so polycultural and non-linear in its incorporation of time: the 1870s–1880s, the mystical past, the present, and the future. *Li Keur* is dramatic (spoken and sung), framed with an overarching metanarrative told by a twenty-first-century grandmother (or grandfather, depending upon casting), and a teenage grandchild. I have written a story within a story that focuses on the 1870s and 1880s within a mystical story. Players sometimes break the fourth wall, particularly the Four Black Geese of Fate, two fiddlers and two dancer/singers, that embody several characters and morph, torment, tantalize, and tease throughout the work. To break the fourth wall, they enter the audience, the orchestra, and interact with the conductor, symphony musicians, and audience members.

Li Keur, how it was made, and how it exists, and how I conceptualize or envision the work, may perhaps challenge the formal classical music hierarchies: "I am the conductor, the artistic director, the manager, the lead violinist, etc." I do not see my role as being a librettist and author who hands over the words and then arrives at the theatre on opening night. From its earliest stages of creation, its envisioning, I saw the piece in its entirety. The methodology I adhere to is to gather a collaboration of performers and makers (e.g., digital designers and set designers) to create something much more than a performance. With *Li Keur*, I present the "we" and propose the "event" is not a performance but an exchange—an offering, perhaps even a ceremony that reaches through time. I perceive performance dates as visits that allow the creation or continuation of relationships rather than the endpoint as a product; this may unnerve conservative sensibilities, along with the ambiguity I present throughout the creation of a work. Further, *Li Keur* breaks or manipulates the familiar of the Eurocentric, classical music tradition. What differentiates

Li Keur from some existing works about Riel is that I wrote a non-Eurocentric, non-linear, and non-historically masculinist narrative. From the very opening I stake a claim for the presence of women at the heart of our Indigenous cultures and continent.

To illustrate this, I am including some of dialogue and libretti from the opening act. The 90-minute, three-act work opens with an overture of sorts: music that establishes a dreamlike quality to the piece. Offstage we hear a young woman narrator, Joséphine-Marie, tell a "becoming" story of a great hunter, a woman called Li Gran Chasseuse, who successfully stalks and kills "our universe," the great bison, and from his hide creates the Michif people, and from the glass beads that fall from her lap as she sews our clothing, creates our stars and planets.[10] As this narration unfolds, two mystical choruses of women set the entire opera, singing in two Michifs of how we sew the natural world. Meanwhile, the children's mystic chorus sings the natural world into being. Translations are in square brackets.

Joséphine-Marie [Spoken]

O komawsmen not kryatewr li bon djyu y la fayt not univers, li plu gro buflo di tot li ten. Wild and beautiful. Ipi Li Gran Buffalo carried A Creation in his belly [In A Beginning our Creator, the Good God, made Our Universe, the greatest bull bison of all time, The Great Buffalo]

Two ghost, or ancestor, choruses of women join this narration and sing antiphonally (in two Michifs and Anishinaabemowin) of how they sew and thus create the world:[11]

Women's Chorus 1 (Heritage/Southern Michif)
Kaashki kwaashonaan [We sew]
Lii roozh faroosh [Wild roses,]
Kaashki kwaashonaan [We sew]

> **Women's Chorus 2 (French Michif):**
> On ko di roz savaj [We sew the wild roses]
> avek di sway ipi lii riban Japonaise
> [with silk threads and Japanese ribbons]

The becoming story continues as the male choruses sing the bison hunt. As the drama builds, so too the orchestra increases the tempo. Then, the children's choruses come in and sing the natural world:

Children's Choruses
Li flax bleu, vayr pi di loo bleu, la bish,
li twaayzoon nakamocihk
L'rnawr y pas
Waagosh aazhawash
Blue flax
Omashkooz, li twaayzoon nakamocihk
Ozhaawashkwaa bag wa jii yay wabigoon
Omashkooz
Waagosh aazhawash kaabagwajiiyay mashkosiwan
Nagmo uk binesi wuk
[Blue flax, water blue and green, the elk, the singing birds. The fox crossing through wild grasses. The elk, singing birds]

The men's choruses join the stage. They sing in a chant-like style antiphonally and create the buffalo herd:

Men's Choruses (tutti)
Hoofing rivers, les rivières noir
Shooki pakitatamoo, pakitatamohk
[Black rivers... Heed the quaking earth]

The 1870s world is thus constructed within the opera. Choruses and narrator are joined by one of the leads, the Anishinaabe keeper of the medicines, Marie Serpente, who proclaims one of the major themes of the work—the spiritual and practical work of women at the heart of our culture(s):

Marie Serpente
L'herbe sainte, odorante, fragrante, sweetgrass [Sweetgrass, fragrant]
Wiigashk gogimaandan, minoma-got [The scent of rebirth]
Nitaawigiwin izhimaagot [We make (the world) whole again]

We are then introduced to Josette, the Michif sharpshooter from nineteenth-century St. Boniface. Finally, we meet the Four Black Geese of Fate and Louis Riel, but we only first see Riel at the very end of the opening act, after placing women, children, and the natural world at the heart of the work. It is 1885 and Riel is writing, a cribbage board on the table. Is he in jail awaiting his murder, his illegal execution by what was then the Canadian state? The Four Black Geese of Fate, ambiguous characters (are they human? Birds? Spirits? Provocateurs?) who fight over Riel. They make a deal with him to play a game of cribbage that will decide his fate:

Riel
Cribbage!
Can't you see, I'm fighting for my destiny.

Black Geese
Mais si vous jouez, Riel
vous gagnerez tout
ou vous perdrez tout.
Les enjeux sont élevés
mais c'est maintenant notre tour, Riel,
distribuons les cartes!

[But Riel when you play, you win all, or you lose all. The stakes are high ... but Riel, it's now our turn, deal the cards!]

As the editor Virginia Durksen stated in a 2018 note after a first read through of a draft: "this opening act places the work in the realm of enchantment."[12] In my notes to the composers and performers I wrote:

> We are communing with a mythic presence, those who are literally with us at all times—ghost fiddlers play a Red River jig, and the underlying rhythm throughout the entire work is always the horse gallop—the Métis are, above all, and to this day, a peoples of the horse. This is reflected in our dance, music, and work. The tonality should be modal/Celtic/medieval French, with the crooked forms of Michif music, and the unexpected melodic and rhythmic shifts of our music. The Black Geese fiddlers will battle not only Riel and others, but also the symphony orchestra and the audience (Steele, 2020).

While in the opera we first meet Riel at a decisive moment in 1885, one in which he gambles with the Fates, I was far more interested in writing about Riel's life than his death. And I was interested in the rich culture of those times, the 1870s and 1880s, to which my own Gaudry and Fayant families belong. Then, too, with this work I intentionally set out to flip the narrative, to have a traditional opera or big-hall symphony audience—that is, predominantly wealthy and white—sense what it is to become the "other." In this, I was perhaps engaging in a form of cultural countermapping, a concept I discuss in more detail below.[13] But more importantly, my main impulse was that our story be told for our people and by our people, that we would recognize ourselves at center stage. This work is written first and foremost for our people: *Li Keur* has as only a secondary aim of introducing non-Métis audiences to some of the Indigenous kinship network cultures existing at the heart of the continent for millennia, of which often little is known outside struggle (Nixon, 2018).

Other than the roles of Marie Serpent, who is Anishinaabe, the Englishman, and the Four Black Geese of Fate (who can be newcomer or Indigenous performers), it was a priority for me to have a Métis cast at the 2019 preview performance with the RSO if at all possible. It was imperative that Indigenous peoples be invited to attend. As I looked out at the full house, I saw that perhaps 30% of the audience were Indigenous. Saskatchewan's late Lieutenant Governor, William Thomas Molloy (a treaty negotiator and a great friend to Indigenous peoples) attended, as did many key people from Métis cultural and scholarly communities, including Sherry Farrell Racette, the language knowledge keeper Norman Fleury, Elder and knowledge keeper Rose Richardson, and many more. I wanted *Li Keur* to claim center stage of the big hall in Regina and onward through a linguistic palette of Michifs and Anishinaabemowin (70% of the text), with French and English in subordinate roles and a narrative story in which we could recognize ourselves.

It was important to me to convey the languages of the prairie kinship webs of my mother's people, a poly-cultural and linguistic weaving that was the lifeblood of her times. This is a project of recovery for my family, especially for my late mother, her own mother, her grandmother in diaspora, and my daughter; it is a re-placing of my female kinship at the heart of the continent. As I stated on opening night, "This hall in this city has hosted so many beautiful languages of the world—Italian, French, Spanish, Ukrainian, German and so many more—and now it is time to hear the languages that have existed in your midst for hundreds and thousands of years, and isn't it wonderful!" And so, the audience heard the languages of the grandmothers and grandfathers.[14]

Li Keur is a story that imagines events that took place during Riel's "missing years" of the early 1870s, when he was in exile south of the Medicine Line (the Canadian–American border). It has been speculated he did many things, including trading or acting as a guide. I wanted to imagine those years and not feel compelled to adhere to the little historical text there is. At the heart of the story is the land and the peoples at the center of the continent: "les entrailles" (the guts).[15] But *Li Keur* is also a love story. Viewing it as neither polemic nor tale of victimhood, I set out to write *Li Keur* as an entertainment for our people as much as I set out to create a piece of high art. I was thus preoccupied with Riel's life, his living, rather than his fights, his trial, and his death and absolutely knew I had to write about the women of his time. I wanted this work to celebrate *lii gens libres*, my mother's people, the Métis, and to tell of their extraordinary creativity, fortitude, and love of beauty—in no way did I feel I needed to "teach" with my work.

Major themes of *Li Keur* include the presence of the mystical (the work opens with a ghostly chorus of women ancestors), the price of love and vision, agency and the identity of a people banished to diaspora and refugeehood (seen in the opera as a children's hunger march in the 1880s),[16] and the beauty and challenge of negotiating cultures and the physical geography of a continent literally and figuratively on fire during the mid-nineteenth century. While the story of *Li Keur* came from my imagination, it is grounded in solid scholarly and land-based research; the love affair at the center of this "entertainment" is historically based, but it also performs as a *pro forma* opera trope. How I found the central love story illustrates the serendipity, or perhaps more likely, "guidance" (being directed by the mystical) that I experienced over the course of preparing to write the book and libretti.

In a mysterious and controversial diary located in the North Dakota State Archives, I read of a Métis guide named Baptiste Robideau who wrote poetry, spoke and wrote in several languages, was educated, and who mysteriously appeared and disappeared across the Medicine Line, clearly politically involved—some speculate this is Riel in his "missing years." And while I expected to learn about Robideau/Riel and his adventures, I was fascinated to read of a central love affair in the diary. An Englishman that Robideau had been hired to guide through the buffalo hunt and the territories watched the love affair between Robideau and a young woman develop, but it was obvious as I read the diary that its author was also falling in love with her and was very jealous of the young woman's affection for Robideau. The young Métis woman's name was Josette.[17] Reading of the love triangle at the heart of the 700-page diary, I knew I had found the central dramatic narrative for my story, with so many of the familiar elements of opera: jealousy, envy, love, lust, adventure, secrets, runaways, and much more.

From the beginning of this project, I always knew that Riel's marriage to Marguerite Monet dit Bellehumeur, daughter of the buffalo hunt (to whom I am related), would not be at the center of the new work; I felt I could not do Marguerite's story justice. Others, such as Métis choreographer Yvonne Chartrand, had already explored Marguerite's life beautifully through dance. Instead, I wanted to focus on a love affair that had never been identified as related to Riel. And, as the events took place in Riel's "missing years," I realized could take some liberties in embroidering and beading the story.

The work is written in six languages—two Michifs, Anishinaabemowin, French, English, and some Latin (if we count the priests blessing the buffalo hunts)—with 70% of the text in Indigenous languages. Working alongside Michif and Anishinaabe partners on *Li Keur* allowed me to present an aurality, a worldview of the grandmothers through syntax, imagery, and especially Anishinaabemowin's gorgeous open vowels (surely a singer's pleasure).[18] The following passage from the "Mending" aria illustrates the negotiation of aesthetic translation by Anishinaabemowin speakers Debra Beach Ducharme and Donna Beach, who work in the medical and educational fields, respectively (and how interesting that the aria is sung by a knowledge keeper of the medicines, a teacher). In this scene, one of the main characters, Marie Serpente, a knowledge keeper of medicines, is called upon to attend to boxers who have gone too far in a match at a meeting of two buffalo brigades, for such competitions were very much a part of the hunt. The men have injured each other badly. As Marie takes out her sinew and needles and begins to bind the men's wounds, she sings the following from the "What Strange Mending is This, of the Violence of Men" aria:

Ni mayagenimaak, [I find it strange]
Ni naaitoon ka ki inaapininde [I repair his wound]
Taa pi skoo makode nanaaitoan [Just like I sew a dress]

After consulting with Elders, the translators took my poetic imagery and syntax, and after we discussed the sense of the passage, they found a way of translating it into something new, yet something retaining the integrity of the original; "I find it strange [that]/ I repair his wound/ Just like I sew a dress."[19]

My goal with *Li Keur*, then, is to flip the sense of "other" for a typical mainstage audience member by presenting a linguistic soundscape more familiar to the 1870s at the heart of the continent. To hear others' languages, to listen closely, can be the beginning of empathy; so too is learning how translators do their work, especially beginning to understand the aesthetics of their languages and cultures as they translate from the aesthetics of my poetic imagery and text. The work illustrates my interest in or rather preoccupation with form: I disassemble or manipulate form as the work tells me to.

Yet I wonder how it might be, that I, daughter of Eilleen, granddaughter of Joséphine Marie Gaudry, could possibly inherit any Métisness, given that my grandmother had gone so deep into whiteness (pink face powder and a parasol in summer lest her skin turn too brown); she was "hidden in plain view" as Susan Sleeper-Smith observes of nineteenth-century Indigenous-French women (2021). This was for sheer survival; her family histories were buried in the heartless, racist twentieth century. She never told us who we are, although we now know she went "home" to see her large Métis family. And yet, for most of my life I lived the life of an ambiguously brown girl, an outsider mistaken by others in a phenomenon my daughter labels their game of ethnic roulette as our being Portuguese, Italian, Greek, Southeast Asian, Persian, Afghani, Lebanese (any Middle Eastern group, actually), Israeli, Indigenous (multiple), or French (close!)—but never Métis. I was 30 years old before I began to unravel some secrets of my family: that for generations we had been Métis people living in St. Vital, Willowbunch, Saint François Xavier, and the Cypress Hills of Montana, and that a few of the grandmothers from the late eighteenth century were Anishinaabe, Sarcie, and probably Nakoda, or—as the census bluntly indicates—"Indian." Through meeting cousins like Randy Gaudry of Willowbunch, Saskatchewan, and Berna-Dean Holland and Sue Nagy of Alberta and Donna McGinnis (all Gaudrys), I have learned that our family spoke numerous languages and that one of the grandfathers translated for Sitting Bull. I learned that we navigated, were entrepreneurs, horsepeople, rodeo contestants, travelers, seamstresses, fiddlers, jiggers, and artists in beads and hides, especially our great-grandmother Marie, who was a beautiful and capable bead worker.[20] But this enormous family was scattered like prairie windflowers after 1885.

And now, it appears, my *modus operandi/vivendi* in the cultural landscape of the twenty-first century is to navigate, to translate, to innovate, to adapt, to make something oddly old yet at the same time new as I try to gather us home. As I do the work I do—spin stories of threads from history and imagination—I now wonder how much of what I do is actually what my people have always done. I recall one day in an army camp in my work as an official Canadian war artist (2008–2010), the first poet to do so, a soldier saying to me, "You are doing what your people have always done; you translate us for civilians."[21] Certainly, in the war requiem I wrote with composer Jeffrey Ryan, *Afghanistan: Requiem for a Generation* (2012), I used some of the traditional Latin text, but I also wrote in the soldiers' vernacular, using the glorious "f-word" in a classical music libretto: I stripped down the Catholic mass for the dead to its essence, then added a text filled with images, story, and voices; working closely with the composer, I sometimes advised him on musical textures and even rhythmic motifs (such as the Morse Code S-O-S in the "Dies Irae").[22] Curiously, I did not see the Métisness embedded in Jeff Ryan and my war requiem, in its form, its deployment of voices, or its imagery until years later. This astonishes me: for heaven's sake, the opening of the requiem is a prayer to the winter solstice, the baritone is a Métis non-commissioned officer (with PTSD), there are wolf track references throughout the libretto, and the raven/blackbird appears throughout, notably with the children's chorus who, as in *Li Keur*, create and embody the natural world. Still, I did not realize how culturally embedded my familial notions were. Now I know better.

I am tempted to write about the occasional exhaustion of working with a type of fragility found in the hierarchy of the classical music world, especially as Canadian cultural institutions are mandated to navigate new ways of working within the context of reconciliation, something that has become obvious specifically when funding opportunities come into play.[23] I have stopped reassuring collaborators when they confront their privilege, their fragility in my presence, however, because it is simply too exhausting, and I believe we are all responsible for making things better. I could write of the amount of emotional energy, the amount of emotional labor that this work entails (because everything I do is peer reviewed by my community)—energy I would rather expend on pure creation—or I could write, perhaps, of a sense I have sometimes that I am expected to show gratitude for having my work performed. But I stand by the quality of my work. And perhaps, tangential to all of this, I could write of sexism and the privileging of composers at the expense of the storyteller, the librettist, the envisioner, but I suppose this is changing, perhaps.[24]

Unwittingly, when I began to research, vision, and write a Riel story in 2017, I now realize that I began a project of cultural "unmapping" or "countermapping," to borrow from critical geography, anthropology, and Indigenous studies (Hunt & Stevenson, 2016). This concept identifies and works to address "the struggle of and over geography [that] remains one of the most significant issues facing Indigenous and nonIndigenous [sic] relations in Canada. Competing claims to territory, borders and boundaries ..." (Hunt & Stevenson, 2016, p. 3). Intuitively, I countermapped the dominant cultural script of focusing on Riel's death and masculinist histories by shifting to a centrality of love and the mystical. Conceptually, the case of Indigenous digital countermapping thus offers an analogy for me: with *Li Keur* I subconsciously—yet sometimes deliberately if I am honest—countermap within the classical music culture and industry. I insisted that we search for and secure a predominantly Métis cast of singers, fiddlers, and choruses and thus was staking a physical, aural (70% Indigenous languages, with French and English in subordinate roles), and cultural claim at center stage in the heart of the continent—a place I consider to already belong to us, yet one we have been shut out of for over 150 years.[25] [26]

And while I worked in a European form and with a sonic palette that could be deemed as informed by the European, it was always my *modus operandi* to disrupt the form and to disrupt the orchestra, literally and figuratively. This disruption comes in the guise of the main fiddler, Alex Kusturok, who breaks the fourth wall of soloist performer or actor on stage and throughout the performance torments, antagonizes, or challenges the orchestra and conductor; the mystical Four Black Geese of Fate sometimes join him in this endeavor. Again, I observe the intersection of my work with Indigenous countermapping of geographies as articulated by Hunt and Stevenson:

> Within countermapping practices, at least some element of the dominant mapping practice is likely to be employed, even if only to be subverted; if counter-mapping practices are not legible according to dominant vocabularies and reading practices, they may not be effective in the way the counter-cartographers desire. (2016, p. 2).

Is my work then a project of subversion? Consciously no, but probably yes. How I created it tells the story.

To begin the work, I felt it necessary to do primary research on the land to listen for what story needed to be told. In 2017, I took a 10,000 km trek with Ella Speckeen (my daughter and traditional Métis fiddler), Jeff Hilberry (her guitarist and my spouse), and Matthew Lloyd, a UK naturalist. Along the way, we inhaled the good air of Montana, swam the Missouri, climbed the buffalo jump near Great Falls, Montana, visited St. Peters where Riel had taught, ate *li galette* in St. Boniface, Manitoba, travelled and visited at the John Arcand Fiddle Festival, and meandered throughout Northern Saskatchewan, Manitoba, and southern Alberta. Along the way we met Métis people, Indigenous people, and many who were "friends" to us (I prefer this to the term "allies"), including the late historian Nicholas Vrooman. I did primary research in museums and archives: in the North Dakota State Archives I read diaries from the 1870s and beyond, in St. Boniface I read the Riel papers at the Centre de Patrimoine, and I did an enormous amount of research with secondary sources.[27] My collaborator, Neil Weisensel, remarked more than a few times that he had never seen so much research done by the librettists of any of his previous projects.[28]

Writing this work, visioning it, and working cross-culturally, especially with legacy institutions such as symphonies and from within the classical music hierarchy, have been and continues to be challenging experiences. But the gifts, the real gifts for me along the way, have been the many relationships forged with so many, with all the people I met on the 10,000 km research journey, and especially with our translators and the singers who breathe life into my words, my narrative of the heart of the great North American continent, and into Weisensel and Kusturok's music. I am most grateful for our people and friends, amazing people such as the Elder and knowledge keeper, Rose Richardson, who has helped through her continuous and peaceable support; another who has accompanied me is the choreographer for *the Li Keur*, the Métis knowledge keeper of dance Yvonne Chartrand (our Elder-in-training!).

As I noted above, I believe that *Li Keur* is a grand visit. I recall hearing Maria Campbell in a radio interview with Carol Off, after the publication of the new edition of her breakthrough work, *HalfBreed*. In the interview, Campbell states that "change is through arts, change is through storytelling, it's through singing songs, it's people visiting each other and talking, it's theatre, it's all of those things" (2019).

Indeed.

Story. Visit. Slow, change. Slowly, walk. Sing, laugh. Until we dance home, again.

Notes

1 These include several productions based on Chester Brown's graphic novel, *Riel: a Comic-Strip Biography* (2003), by Persephone Theatre, Infiniti Theatre, and Théâtre La Chapelle, *Riel, a Comic Strip Stage Play* (2016), a Festivale de Castellier shadow puppet production of *Louis Riel: Une Bande Dessinée*, (2016), John Coulter's *The Trial of Louis Riel* (1967), Musicalmania's *Hey Riel*, with Jocelyn Ladouceur as guest jigger (2020), Jean Louis Roux's *Bois-Brûlés, reportage épique sur Louis Riel* (2017), Ryan Gladstone's, and *The Seven Lives of Louis Riel* (2009). Recently, women have begun to tell the Riel story, or the story of the Métis and First Nations women around Riel. These include Métis choreographer Yvonne Chartrand and Russian-born Ania Storoszczuk's dance production, *Marguerite* (2000), based on the life of Marguerite Monet dit Bellehumeur Riel, and Francis Koncan's *Women of the Fur Trade* (2020).

2 The other two reviewers are Eugene Walz, Department of English (Film Studies), University of Manitoba, and Diane Payment, Parks Canada, Winnipeg. Payment writes of the production: "Women may have played a largely supportive role in the 19th century but why must we persist in depicting them merely as irrational creatures or sexual objects."

3 I didn't see the 2017 *Louis Riel*, but it was reported by Métis colleagues and cultural knowledge keepers in attendance that the 2017 version failed on multiple counts and was insulting to many. In a November 5, 2022, email to me, Nicole Stonyk remarks, "2017—the beginning of creating an entirely new narrative surrounding Louis Riel and others who are desperately trying to recycle arguably the most racist and pan-Indigenous musical representation of Louis Riel and Indigenous People in Canadian history." Jean Teillet notes that "the opera and its content, which stumbled from beginning to

end over its crude portrayal of Riel, the colonial bias, and the offensive stereotypes. Riel is portrayed as an insane, francophone, megalomaniac mystic. Prime Minister John A. Macdonald and Georges-Étienne Cartier are cartoons. Chief Pound maker is a noble savage. The priests are moral compasses. The Métis women are cardboard cutouts of mother, wife, and sister. The Indian men are silent drunks, and the Indian women are prostitutes" (2018, p. 30).

4 "You referred to Neil as a 'newcomer.' I really like how you avoid the 'settler' terminology so commonly used today. Emma LaRoque commented on avoiding the term 'settler' during the [Mawachihotaak] conference. That using the term 'settler' implies Indigenous peoples were 'unsettled' as noble savages in an untamed wilderness" (N. Stonyk, personal communication, November 6, 2022).

5 Indeed, "madness" is a favorite trope of many Riel productions and commentaries, one which I did not adhere to in my book or libretti.

6 I tend to eschew the terminology of postcolonial theory, which I find can be reductive or restrictive and frequently used without nuance.

7 Neil and I wish to thank our colleague, Vic Froese, head of the library at Canadian Mennonite University for help in designing this project, as well as research assistants Bryna Link (Peguis Indigenous) and Hannah Connolly, both of whom worked diligently on this project, as well as all our translators.

8 Whenever I speak in public about reconciliation, I always caution the impatient: "Have patience, it took 400 plus years to get here so it is not going to take four years or even forty years to complete the reconciliation project!"

9 Conducted by Gordon Gerrard, the cast included Riva Farrell Racette (narrator), Jordan Daniels (fiddler); Rebecca Cuddy (Josette), Melanie Courage (soprano roles, including Marie Serpent and Marguerite Riel), James Westman (Riel/Robideau), James McLelland (Black Geese of Fate/Englishman), Marion Newman (Black Geese of Fate roles), the RSO, and a Métis chorus conducted and directed by the late Dominic Gregorio, who tragically left for the spirit world the same week as rehearsals began. His chorus performed with full hearts.

10 Out of respect I did not want to adapt or borrow any creation stories and thus wrote a becoming story.

11 Sherry Farrell Racette's 2004 doctoral dissertation, *Sewing Ourselves Together: Clothing, Decorative Arts and the Expression of Metis and Half Breed Identity*, informed my thinking while I was writing the libretti. Coincidentally, her daughter Riva was our narrator for the RSO production.

12 V. Durksen, personal communication, February, 2018. I thank her for this and other valuable insight and observations.

13 I wish to thank my colleague, Dillon Apsassin, one of our research assistants on the Red River Jig Network (www.redriverjig.com), for introducing me to countermapping.

14 It was not lost on me for one minute that the rehearsal and performance period was in Regina, the city in which Riel was murdered.

15 From the *Collected Works of Louis Riel*. In his journals of 1885 Riel writes, "L'Esprit de Dieu m'a fait voir un quart plein de marchandises. Sur le fond du Quart étaient écrites les paroles suivantes: 'Les entrailles du Nord.' O mon Dieu! Accordez-moi, la grâce de conquérir le

Nord et de Maîtriser tout ce qu'il a: donnez-moi les entrailles du nord" (1985, p. 387). Translation by S. M. Steele: "The Spirit of God showed me a crate full of merchandise. On the bottom of it were the words, 'The heart of the North.' O my God! For the love of Jesus, Mary, Joseph, and St. John the Baptist, grant me the grace to conquer the North and to master all within it: give me the heart of the North."

16 Written during the Syrian refugee crisis, I saw many parallels with the Métis experience of the 1880s.
17 Heather Devine located the diary and proposed the link to Riel. After hearing an interview with her on the CBC, I decided to go to North Dakota myself, where I downloaded and read the diary. I have located a Josette, a contemporary of Sara Riel, in the school records of the Grey Nuns in St. Boniface but have not been able to substantiate that she is the same Josette as in the diary.
18 The translators of the *Li Keur* text are as follows: Verna de Montigny (Traditional/Southern Michif); Jules Chartrand, June Bruce, Lorraine Coutu, and Agathe Chartrand (St Laurent French Michif); and Donna Beach and Debra Beach Ducharme (Anishinaabemowin).
19 The Anishinaabemowin translators told me that translating this work enhanced their language abilities (D. Beach-Ducharme and D. Beach, personal communication, August, 2018).
20 My great-grandmother Marie Fayant (1886–1969) was perhaps Nakoda, possibly adopted by the Fayants, a Métis family. She remains a mystery to us, despite some of my cousins having met her many times when they were young, long before some Métis families talked about their genealogies. One of the mysteries is that Marie Fayant's birth certificate indicates her parents' as being in their mid-50s. This leads us to believe Marie was adopted; that, and the fact she was very "brown," perhaps the most "Indian" of our very "French" family, and perhaps adopted during one of the famines of the late 19th century in Montana.
21 Corporal T. Scott, personal communication, May, 2009.
22 Alas, despite the form and text chosen and written by me and the requiem being based on my lived experience as a Canadian war artist who went to Afghanistan, and that I chose the composer to work with my text, *Afghanistan: Requiem for a Generation* remains known as composer Jeff Ryan's war requiem. This in no way reflects Jeff's collegiality or point of view; rather it reflects the inflexibility of the classical music industry and hierarchy.
23 In her preface to *Writing the Circle: Native Women of Western Canada*, Emma Larocque writes: "unlike many white intellectuals, we were not born into our stations in life" (1990, xxii). I might add that of my generation, some were not born to nor could have aspired to achieve stations in the musical hierarchy—as long as artistic directors, conductors, and critics (paradoxically, some performing "allyship" in the public space) continued to exoticize, ignore, or erase the Métis voice and, importantly, our approach to co-creation and envisioning. As an aside, my great-aunt Elizabeth Robinson's poetry and her account of residential school can be found in *Writing the Circle*.
24 Dylan Robinson's compelling *Hungry Listening: Resonant Theory for Indigenous Sound Studies* (2020) is an excellent start to this conversation, although the role of sexism in the music industry should also be factored in.
25 If Métis performers were unavailable for Métis roles, I stated that we should search outward in a radiant practice; for example, beginning with what Anishinaabe or Oji-Cree performers were available and then casting further afield if we must.

26 As Quinn Bell writes in the March 17, 2019, review of the RSO performance: "In making and performing this unique Canadian opera, it is hoped that audiences will again learn to embrace the cultural and linguistic complexity that once thrived here, in a time when English was very much the minority tongue. The syllables and sounds of the Michif and Saulteaux, of the Fransaskois and Francomanitobain [sic], are beautiful. These are functional languages and should be protected for future generations."
27 A bibliography is available upon request.
28 One thing I did not do was read the score of or listen to the 1967 Riel opera, save for a brief scan of the first few pages of the score at the Canadian Music Centre near my home in Vancouver. I wanted to get a taste of what Moore and Somers had written and nothing more.

References

Bell, Q. (2019, March 17). "RSO celebrates Riel's legacy." *The Carrilon*. https://www.carillonregina.com/rso-celebrates-riels-legacy/

Campbell, M. (2019, November 29). *On the pain and relief of re-releasing Halfbreed with uncut account of RCMP rape* [Radio broadcast]. Canadian Broadcasting Corporation. https://www.cbc.ca/radio/asithappens/as-it-happens-friday-edition-1.5378245/mariacampbell-on-the-pain-and-relief-of-re-releasing-halfbreed-with-uncut-account-of-rcmprape-1.5378256

Farrell Racette, S. (2004). *Sewing ourselves together: Clothing, decorative arts and the expression of Metis and half breed identity* [Doctoral dissertation, University of Manitoba]. https://mspace.lib.umanitoba.ca/xmlui/handle/1993/3304

Giroux, M. (2018). The Goddamn Opera is Dead! *Canadian Notes and Queries*. http://notesandqueries.ca/essays/the-goddamn-opera-is-dead/

Globe and Mail. (2002, November 23). Diary found by historian may clear up Riel mystery. https://www.theglobeandmail.com/news/national/diary-found-by-historian-may-clear-up-riel-mystery/article1028367

Harris, R. (2017, April 21). Grand visions flame out at Louis Riel opera. *Globe and Mail*. https://www.theglobeandmail.com/arts/theatre-and-performance/theatre-reviews/grand-visions-flame-out-at-louis-riel-opera/article34779237/

Hunt, D., & Stevenson, S. A. (2016). Decolonizing geographies of power: Indigenous digital counter-mapping practices on Turtle Island. *Settler Colonial Studies*, 7(3), 1–21. https://doi.org/10.1080/2201473X.2016.1186311

LaRocque, E. "Preface." (1990). In A. Perreault & S. Vance (eds.), *Writing the circle: Native women of Western Canada* (pp. xv–xxx). NeWest Publishers.

Nixon, L. (2018). *Prairie families: Cree-Métis-Saulteux materialities as Indigenous feminist materialist record of kinship-based selfhood* [Master's thesis, Concordia University]. https://spectrum.library.concordia.ca/id/eprint/984472/

Teillet, J. (2018). The sermon from the mount: The messages in the Canadian Opera Company's remount of the Riel opera. *University of Toronto Quarterly*, 87(4), 29–36. https://doi.org/10.3138/utq.87.4.04

Riel, L. (1985). *Les Éditions Complètes de Louis Riel/The Collected Works of Louis Riel*. G. F. Stanley, R. J. A. Huel, G. Martel, T. Flanagan, & G. Campbell (Eds.). The University of Alberta Press.

Robinson, Dylan. (2020). *Hungry listening: Resonant theory for Indigenous sound studies*. University of Minnesota Press.

Simeonov, J. (2017, April 27). Discomfort: Louis Riel at the COC. *Schmopera*. https://www.schmopera.com/discomfort-louis-riel-at-the-coc/

Sleeper-Smith, S. (2001). *Indian women and French men: Rethinking cultural encounter in the western Great Lakes*. University of Massachusetts Press.

Steele, S., with Weisensel, N., Link, B., Froese, V., & Connolly, H. (n.d.) *Li Keur Indigenous Translation Database*. Canadian Mennonite University. https://omeka.cmu.ca/s/Riel-Heart-of-the-North/page/welcome1 (accessed 4 January 2023).

Walz, E., Payment, D., & Laroque, E. (1981). Review: Three views of Riel. *Manitoba History*, 1. www.mhs.mb.ca/docs/mb_history/01/threeviewsofriel.shtml

· 1 1 ·

MÉTIS ARTS AS EDUCATION: VISUAL STORYTELLING, AND MORE, IN ALBERTA

Yvonne Poitras Pratt and Billie-Jo Grant

Métis Arts as Education: Visual Storytelling and More in Alberta

Over the years, Métis voices and perspectives in the Alberta curriculum have been silenced, vilified, or misrepresented, as in other provinces and territories across the lands now known as Canada (Forsythe, 2021; Paulson et al., 2015; Poitras Pratt, 2021). This concerning and negligent stance persists despite the rich, compelling history and contemporary presence of Métis people throughout the province. In 2012, the Métis Nation of Alberta took a much-needed step toward reclaiming our voice in education by transferring its education mandate from the provincial organization to its affiliate, the Rupertsland Institute, which has historically focused its efforts on training for the labor market. In 2015, the education staff of one increased to four, supported by the volunteer efforts of six members of the Alberta Métis Education Council (Poitras Pratt & Lalonde, 2019). This small team of educators working at Rupertsland has realized several key educational initiatives: the co-creation of foundational knowledge themes with Métis community members, an emerging Michif language initiative, and growing efforts to support early childhood learning. These activities have served to complement and enrich the overall teaching and learning experiences of K–12 educators across Alberta while shifting the perspectives of fellow Albertans.

Alongside these sorely needed contributions developed and advanced by Rupertsland education staff, a number of educational initiatives have been created and developed by fellow Métis educators and respected community members who are invested in and supportive of our self-determining moves in education. In Alberta, some of these initiatives have been developed by community members who have recognized the need to educate the wider public about the Métis,[1] while other educator-led initiatives have been targeted for K–12 impact and inclusion. Each of these activities takes a slightly different approach and considers a different audience, but they all share a common vision: educating our own and others about the Métis. What is obvious when looking across these varied examples is that the arts are an effective avenue for inviting both those who wish to learn more and those who are surprised that there is more to learn.

As professional educators, we argue that it is essential to move beyond the initial lure of artistic expression into critical engagement with the topic of interest. In other words, there is a process of creating teaching and learning resources that signals ethical and decolonizing engagement. This happens at both the individual and community levels:

> For curriculum to reach beyond the colonial historical context, educators must first engage in critical self-examination, and then seek active input on learning material from Indigenous community members to respectfully engage in this work. These factors ensure authentic learning around Indigenous perspectives is taking place despite the current lack of pathways into the realm of reconciliation (Poitras Pratt & Lalonde, 2019, para. 2).

This chapter focuses on two aesthetically inclined initiatives that supplement the central offerings created by the Rupertsland education team that demonstrate a respectful and reciprocal arrangement between Métis community members and Métis educators: the *Métis Voices* digital storytelling project (www.metisvoices.ca/) and the *Métis Memories of Residential School and Other Colonial Schooling* mural mosaic and art card project (www.muralmosaic.com/metis-memories/). The first project advances the digital storytelling work undertaken in the Fishing Lake Métis Settlement in 2009–2011 (Poitras Pratt, 2020), while the mosaic art card project builds on survivor stories contained in the *Métis Memories of Residential Schools* (2004). Together, these projects represent a promising return to a *collective* approach by bringing authentic Métis community voices and stories into Alberta's classrooms by drawing on the power of arts and media agency. These projects, envisioned as supportive of K–12 educators and professional teaching standards (see Alberta Education, Teaching Quality Standard 5), are also helping to build a bridge between academic knowledge and Indigenous knowledge traditions. With demand for authentically Indigenous—in this case Métis—resources growing across the province, this chapter sets out some promising practices to consider as similar initiatives are imagined and brought into K–12 classrooms.

For those of us of Métis ancestry, the reminder of our collective worldviews and cultural traditions is important (Alberta Education, 2005; Campbell, 2010). As professional educators, one working in the K–12 realm and the other in a post-secondary context, we are cognizant that we operate within a Western system of schooling where hierarchical structures and competitive natures dominate (Battiste, 2013; Poitras Pratt & Gladue, 2021). We are also acutely aware and regularly reminded that colonialism has had a significant and lasting impact on the ways in which our people think about themselves and how they have adopted certain practices to survive in a post-1885 world (Adams, 1975; Campbell, 1972; Cardinal, 1976; LaRocque, 1975, 2010; Teillet, 2019). Our professional and personal lives are deeply intertwined, and we recognize that it is next to impossible to separate what we do on a professional level with how we live and operate in our everyday lives. This is not to be viewed as a negative; it simply is. What we have both found is that the arts provide a creative and nurturing way to restore our spirits, to stay afloat, and to keep our passion for what is often an intense and demanding work life alive and well (Klopper, 2014). In many ways, the arts represent a sustaining force in the frequently difficult work we undertake on a daily basis. The arts also serve as an engaging and accessible bridge for drawing on community-led initiatives to create rich educational resources with appropriate principles upheld and professional expectations set out.

How the Arts Serve Métis Community Interests

The arts are slowly but steadily gaining recognition for their ability to sustain and support Indigenous people's needs; over the years, they have been valued for their life-sustaining role in health and wellbeing (Cardinal-Schubert, 1999; Ryan, 1999; van Styvendale et al., 2021); and, in recent times, they have shown signs of a promising role in education (Akinleye, 2021; Davis, 2018; Heckenberg, 2018; Irwin & Farrell, 1996). However the arts are imagined or deployed, it is "the processes through which local, subaltern communities 'take hold' of literacy" (McCarty, 2005, p. 1) to make it their own that is of particular interest in the work we do. McCarty's *Language, Literacy, and Power in Schooling* demonstrates the ways in which Indigenous peoples are using the arts to

> wedge open new spaces of possibility—alternatives to an either-or, unilingual, and monoculturalist divide. Informed by insiders—those who often are the targets of standardizing regimes ... show the emancipatory potentials that arise when local literacies are claimed and appropriated for local ends. (p. 2).

In an inspiring turn of phrase, these creative acts are now viewed by Indigenous communities and scholars as "art for life's sake" (van Styvendale et al., 2021) rather than the dominant understanding of art as a leisure pursuit or a subject for only the most refined tastes.

The Métis have integrated arts into their daily lives, honoring and following their First Nation ancestral ways while also creating their own unique art forms along the way. As Cheryl Troupe and Lawrence Barkwell (2006) describe it in their chapter on Métis decorative arts in *Métis Legacy II*, "Métis artistic expression ... is a delicate blend of European and First Nations art forms, materials, and techniques blended in a creative synthesis to meet not only the Métis' utilitarian needs but also [to] display a sense of self-identity and nationhood" (p. 104). The arts, of course, have a multitude of expressions: visual, print, performance, dance, and music, among others. In our own arts-based practices, we draw primarily on visual arts traditions with a complement of multimedia formats. Our educational arts-based practices are intended to support and empower Métis voices and perspectives and to educate others about the Métis through purposeful sharing. We concur with Rita Irwin and Ruby Farrell (1996), who once noted that arts education from an Indigenous perspective is "one area of study in which people come together to learn about, and from, one another"; we are also in agreement with these authors that "it is better to raise questions in an effort to begin the process of understanding than it is to remain naive about the questions" (p. 73).

In contemporary times, the Métis have taken up the power of the written word in a substantive way to reclaim and restore their side of the colonial story in what was once referred to as resistance literature (Adams, 1972; Campbell, 1972, 2018; Teillet, 2019). As Métis scholar and matriarch Emma LaRocque

(2010) muses, perhaps Indigenous people "have had about enough of enduring, we are moving to take our places in Canadian society as socially and culturally vibrant intellectuals and artists without the cultural burdens of misrepresentations and marginalization" (p. 170). The intellectual contributions of Métis scholars and educators, when viewed through a stance of perpetual victimhood, risk being narrowly slotted into an "aesthetics of healing" rather than being valued for their intrinsic value (LaRocque, 2010, p. 168).

One of the better-known Métis artists of our time, Christi Belcourt, has written on how Métis identity is expressed through the arts:

> We are as resilient as a weed and as beautiful as a wildflower.... Resilience is the capacity to recover and cope with adversity. Resistance is a struggle against oppression. [Christi Belcourt] sees plants as metaphors for Métis resilience. (Farrell Racette, 2011, p. 7)

Throughout the years, the "Métis are people who have always had strong traditional values on the subject of education for their children. These ideals were seriously altered with the introduction of the residential school system" (Logan, 2001, p. 61). In the revised edition of *Stories of the Road Allowance People*, Métis Elder Maria Campbell (2010) shares stories of the old ones and pays homage to contemporary Indigenous artist Sherry Farrell Racette, "who loved the stories and gave them life through her art" (2011, p. 5). In this translation of oral traditions into print and visual imagery, we witness how the arts bring an enlivened sense of who we are in a world that is either unaware of or confused by our complex identity. In 1999, Leah Dorion and Darren Préfontaine wrote, "American and Canadian scholars have documented a whole tradition of racist literary works which stereotyped the Métis people. *Rarely did Métis people write about themselves*" (p. 25, emphasis added). In an art exhibition pamphlet that accompanied *Resilience / Resistance, Métis Art (1880–2011)*, the inclusion of the following passage in a Parks Canada (2011) publication is further evidence of how this confusion persists today:

> One of the questions we have received at Batoche in the past was whether or not the Métis community still existed or if there were any Métis who still lived in the area. While many Canadians may know elements of Métis history, not all have a strong awareness of contemporary Métis society and culture. (p. 4)

A 2016 federally commissioned report puts the matter directly:

> Notwithstanding this history, the Métis have largely been forgotten until recent years in the historical narrative as a distinct rights-bearing Aboriginal people. Part of this challenge has been the Métis unique heritage and history and because they have not, as a people, fit into an easily identifiable legal box. (Issac, 2016, p. 3)

It is in this confusing context of misunderstanding and lack of awareness that we make the case for why Métis arts can serve as education for our own people and for others.

Bridging and Integrating Métis Arts into the Classroom

As educators who are committed to decolonizing, Indigenizing, and reconciliatory aims in our professional roles, we are keenly aware that the arts provide powerful avenues for learning and teaching. We are also aware that the arts can be perceived as a superficial pastime in which deep learning and critical engagement with ideas do not readily come to mind (Sensoy & DiAngelo, 2011). By sharing our community-based projects, we are pulling aside the curtains to offer an insider's look into how the Métis community thinks and talks about the use of the arts as a tool for social change.

Yvonne: In 2009, I made the decision to return to my parents' ancestral community, the Fishing Lake Métis Settlement in northeastern Alberta, to dedicate my doctoral work in service of community needs (Poitras Pratt, 2020). In wanting to focus specifically on the Métis, I had two ideas to offer to the community: either photovoice or digital storytelling. Suzi Barthel and Ryck, my main contact in the community and its political leader, respectively, were both adamant that it had to be digital stories. Fortunately, my mother and I had taken part in a digital storytelling workshop a few months earlier, and our intergenerational story, focused on Tootsie (my maternal grandmother) and her role in the Fishing Lake community, was projected on a blank wall for the room of Elders who had made space for us in the seniors lodge. As soon as the story started playing, the room came alive; the group started to recognize some of the people in the historical photos and the names of places they knew well—these were familiar people, places, and stories. As the energy in the room shifted from curiosity to excitement, I knew the time was right to pitch my idea: what would they think of making their own digital stories? My friend Suzi, who had organized the meeting, grabbed a tattered print book from the coffee table and waved it in front of the group: "See how these books fall apart after a while—these digital stories will remain forever if we take good care of them!" The group was largely convinced so I lingered in the space after we were done the formal part of the sharing, tidying up the room and answering questions from some of the quieter attendees. I will always remember one question: "But Yvonne, I don't read or write; how can I do this?" And her reaction, after I reassured her that this wasn't an issue with a format that privileged voice, photos, and the inclusion of Michif or Cree, was equally memorable—she started to cry and stated, "No one has ever said that to me." I felt that the fact that I was Métis and my family were community members they knew and recognized made it possible for some of the inevitable distrust of outsiders in this tiny community to dissolve and, more importantly, for the embers of our storytelling traditions to start burning again (Poitras Pratt, 2022). Since then, I have worked with members of the Fishing Lake Métis Settlement community to create 19 digital stories that are distinctive in their intergenerational telling and honoring the collective voice, despite their diversity. More recently, I had the privilege of sharing these stories with my friend and colleague Billie-Jo Grant, who immediately saw the value of these stories as authentic and accessible teaching resources. Together, we worked with the original storytellers to create a set of teaching resources based on what the storytellers wanted educators and learners to gain from their stories. These resources are now housed at https://www.metisvoices.ca/.

Billie-Jo: In 2018, I took a leave from teaching inclusive education in K–12 classrooms to work with the Rupertsland Institute. My main focus in this role was to help create foundational knowledge and resources that would ultimately support the teaching of Métis perspectives in the K–12 educational system. It was in this new role that I came across the 2004 book *Métis Residential Schools: A Testament to the Strength of the Métis*. It was evident that the publisher of these heartfelt residential school reflections was the Métis Nation of Alberta but as there was no name on the book, I remained curious as to who had compiled these stories so respectfully. Since the learning around residential schools is so deeply personal for me in my professional role, I valued how this book demonstrated integrity in its sharing. I asked around and was given contact information for Jude D. Daniels, who informed me that she and a co-author had crafted the book, working closely with survivors.

My mind was churning with the possibilities. I had a vision for a teaching resource but no idea how it would come to fruition. I worked with my trusted colleague and good friend, Yvonne Poitras Pratt, to find ways to support this work; several years after I found that book, she called to say, "I found a grant!"

Together we sent in a Canadian Heritage Grant, submitting it minutes before the deadline but happily receiving news, months later, that the application had been successful. It was now time to make the dream into a reality. We knew this important work could not be done without the guidance of an Elder, so we reached out to Angie Crerar, a well-respected Métis Elder living in Grande Prairie; we knew she was a residential school survivor and strong community leader who would lead us in a good way. Her involvement and leadership turned out to be even more vital, as the COVID-19 pandemic radically changed how we anticipated engaging with survivors. Our small team eventually consisted of the original author, a Métis Elder and residential school survivor, a teacher educator, and a K–12 specialist educator. We also brought in our own families—our daughters are all artists in their own ways—who contributed their own artistic gifts to the impact of the project. I also reached out to a well-known artist and trusted friend, Lewis Lavoie of Mural Mosaic, whose artistic work involving murals has enjoyed enormous success with learners of all ages from diverse cultures. As Métis people who are passionate about using education to empower our people, we all felt it was important that Lewis would be able to translate this sensitive subject matter into visuals that respectfully and accurately told our truths. To his credit, Lewis listened deeply and asked important questions. If he didn't get it right, Lewis went back to the easel—each and every time, he reassured us that it wasn't about him, it was about getting it right. Many of our early discussions centered on finding an image would bring together the diverse stories represented by the 24 mural mosaic tiles. The original artwork that Samantha, Yvonne's adult daughter, had painted of a sash depicted as a Métis infinity symbol was perfect.

As educators, we knew that the art, while beautiful, was not enough. It was now time to go deeper: including teaching statements, reflective questions, and foundational knowledge on each piece would turn the art cards into valuable teaching and learning resources. The "little project that could" ultimately *did*—it was launched during Métis Week 2021 on an online platform with an audience of residential schools survivors, fellow educators, Métis community members, and the interested public. Since that launch, the project has grown exponentially through multiple presentations; notably, a copy of the print version of our mosaic project was gifted to Pope Francis by Elder Angie Crerar at the Vatican in summer 2022. Knowing that teaching and learning is most valuable when shared, we applied to the Canadian Museum of Human Rights (CMHR), and the results are currently on display in the Community Corridor of the CMHR and in the lobby of the Chateau Laurier Fairmont

Hotel in Winnipeg. A more accessible form of this resource available to all teachers is housed online at https://www.muralmosaic.com/metis-memories/.

Lessons Learned While Integrating Métis Arts into Education

So, what have we learned while doing these community-based artistic projects that have become valuable teaching and learning resources? As Métis people, we are honoring our traditional ways and valuing Indigenous principles by listening to and acting on the wisdom of our ancestors and respected community members. Our collective Métis ways are re-emerging despite the challenges of a society that values individualism, collectivism, and material gain. In recognizing that we, as Métis, have "a personal responsibility to collective survival [that] requires the ability to adapt" (Poitras Pratt, 2020, p. 135), we are respecting our inherent diversity alongside ancestral traditions. As Métis educators working with community members who bring valuable knowledge from their lived experiences, we represent a diverse group of people who are coming together with *shared values* to imagine new ways forward. The ways in which we are learning to bring community-based knowledge traditions into education requires an ethos of respect, reciprocity, sharing, and mutual recognition of our distinctive gifts (Poitras Pratt & Gladue, 2022; Royal Commission on Aboriginal Peoples, 1996; United Nations, 2007). In many ways, we are learning to lift our own people—placing mutual respect, reciprocity, and relationality at the forefront of our collective work.

As exemplified in these projects, the role of educators as a skilled group of professionals who have the requisite expertise to bring Indigenous knowledge traditions into formal learning settings is essential. In turn, Métis knowledge-keepers and Elders are placing their faith and trust in us to represent the Métis nation and its people in the best way possible. Our guiding principle—"braver together"—allows us to collectively envision and create a space for Métis people to have their stories heard in a respectful and empowering way.

Note

1 The Métis Crossing Cultural Heritage Gathering Centre in Smoky Lake, Alberta, is a vivid example of the wider Métis community taking on public education: https://metiscrossing.com/. Another community-led example of drawing on Métis cultural arts and traditions to help educate and inform our own and others is found in southern Alberta at the Hills

are Alive cultural camp event, typically held in the Cypress Hills area each spring: https://m.facebook.com/profile.php?id=100064641281317&eav=AfZoDhmGgOfm1SmFFucB04khmKVrB6C_eQRgn1Qcn1KePqWx-p6cLPBvdLWMkH3FcqU&paipv=0&_rdr. Finally, there is the land-based initiative to reclaim Métis voice and stories is found in

Community Connection Statement

Yvonne Poitras Pratt (Métis Nation of Alberta card 009347) has long been active in the realm of Métis education, serving in 2012–2013 as the first ever Associate Director, Métis Education at the Rupertsland Institute, a Métis Centre of Excellence. Since her recruitment to the Werklund School of Education, Yvonne has maintained close ties to the provincial Métis community through her service on the Alberta Métis Education Council (2015–present) and as an executive member and associate scholar of the Rupertsland Centre for Métis Research (University of Alberta). With ancestry tracing back to the 1600s, some of the more prominent Métis names in her family tree include Poitras, Parenteau, Fayant, and Calliou, with the notable involvement of great-great grandfather Pierre Poitras in the 1869 Provisional Government.

As the former Associate Director of K–12 Education, Billie-Jo's goal is to ensure that strong Métis education is commonplace in our education system and guarantee that Métis are no longer a "forgotten people." Billie-Jo is an active citizen in the Métis Nation of Alberta and raised her three children to be proud Métis individuals. Her Métis ancestry traces back to family roots in northern Saskatchewan (Pruden) and Fraser (Fort Chipewyan), with family connections to the Flett and Courteille names. Additional ancestry traces back to the 1800s and includes Colin Fraser and his Métis wife Nancy Ann Beaudry. Billie-Jo promotes pride in Indigenous identity for all students and works tirelessly to improve educational outcomes and inequities. Billie-Jo is currently the Indigenous consultant with Greater St. Albert Catholic Schools.

References

Alberta Education. (2005). "Indigenous pedagogy: Worldviews and Aboriginal cultures." In *Our words, our ways: Teaching First Nations, Métis and Inuit learners.* https://www.learnalberta.ca/content/aswt/indigenous_pedagogy/documents/worldviews_aboriginal_culture.pdf

Canadian Artists' Representation / Le Front des artistes canadiens (CARFAC). (2021). *Indigenous protocols for the visual arts: A practical guide for navigating the complex world of*

Indigenous protocols for cultural expressions in the visual arts sector. https://static1.squaresp
ace.com/static/61e830a9a1fa890cec5c1521/t/62b0ab66799341026eda23d1/1655745382
945/Indigenous+Protocols+for+the+Visual+Arts.pdf

de Bruin, L. R., Burnard, P., & Davis, S. (Eds.) (2018). *Creativities in arts education, research and practice: International perspectives for the future of learning and teaching.* Brill.

Farrell Racette, S. (2011). Resilience, resistance – Métis art, 1880–2011 / curated by Sherry Farrell Racette. http://parkscanadahistory.com/publications/batoche/metis-art-e-2011.pdf

Forsythe, L. (2021). Becoming the Métis Inclusion Coordinator. In J. MacDonald & J. Markides (Eds.), *Brave Work in Indigenous Education* (pp. 181–186). DIO Press.

Heckenberg, R. (2018). Bunya pine, goanna and star clusters. In L. de Bruin, P. Burnard, & S. Davis (Eds.), *Creativities in Arts Education, Research and Practice* (pp. 67–83). Brill. https://doi.org/10.1163/9789004369603_005

Irwin, R. L., & Farrell, R. (1996). The framing of Aboriginal art. In D. A. Long & O. P. Dickason (Eds.), *Visions of the heart: Canadian Aboriginal issues* (pp. 57–92). Harcourt Brace & Company Canada.

Issac, T. (2016). *A matter of national and constitutional import: Report of the Minister's Special Representative on Reconciliation with Métis.* Technical Report. Indigenous and Northern Affairs Canada. https://publications.gc.ca/collections/collection_2016/aanc-inac/R5-123-2016-eng.pdf

Klopper, C. (2014). The lived experience: Finding joy though working in the arts. In N. Lemon, S. Garvis, & C. Klopper (Eds.), *Representations of working in arts education: Stories of learning and teaching,* pp. 15–28. Intellect Ltd.

Manitowabi, M. C. (n.d.) *Indigenous educational materials.* https://www.marissamanitowabi.net/

McCarty, T. L. (Ed.). (2005). *Language, literacy, and power in schooling.* Taylor & Francis Group.

Métis Nation of Alberta. (2004). *Métis memories of residential schools: A testament to the strength of the Métis.* https://www.muralmosaic.com/metis-memories/

Paulson, J., Poitras Pratt, Y., & Contreras, G. (2015). Métis K-12 education discussion paper. A report commissioned by The Rupertsland Institute, a Métis Centre of Excellence. https://www.rupertsland.org/wp-content/uploads/2017/08/metis-education-k-12-final-march-13-2015.pdf

Poitras Pratt, Y. (2020). *Digital storytelling in Indigenous education: A decolonizing journey for a Métis community.* Routledge.

Poitras Pratt, Y. (2021). Resisting symbolic violence: Métis community engagement in lifelong learning. *International Journal of Lifelong Education,* 40(4), 382–394. https://doi.org/10.1080/02601370.2021.1958017

Poitras Pratt, Y. & Gladue, K. (2022). Re-defining academic integrity with Indigenous truths. In S. Eaton & J. C-Hughes (Eds.), *Academic integrity in Canada: An enduring and essential challenge* (pp. 103–123). https://link.springer.com/chapter/10.1007/978-3-030-83255-1_5

Poitras Pratt, Y., & Lalonde, S. (2019). The Alberta Métis Education Council: Realizing self-determination in education. In S. Carr-Stewart (Ed.), *Knowing the Past, Facing the Future: Indigenous Education in Canada* (pp. 265–287). Purich.

Resilience: 50 Indigenous art cards and teaching guide. (n.d.). https://resilienceproject.ca/

Royal Commission on Aboriginal Peoples. (1996). *Highlights from the Report of the Royal Commission on Aboriginal Peoples.* https://www.rcaanc-cirnac.gc.ca/eng/1100100014597/1572547985018

Sensoy, O., & DiAngelo, R. (2011). *Is everyone really equal? An introduction to key concepts in social justice education.* Teachers College Press.

United Nations. (2008). *United Nations declaration on the rights of Indigenous peoples.* http://www.un.org/esa/socdev/unpfii/documents/DRIPS_en.pdf

· 1 2 ·

RAINDROPS, FIDDLES, AND TALL TALES: NAVIGATING OUR DIVERSITY THROUGH STORYTELLING

Angie Tucker

I wish that I could replay the sounds of a darkening sky rolling into the prairies. A low, deep rumble begins in the distance. The wind picks up so gently at first, and the tall grasses—the hair of Mother Earth—begin to move together in many swirling bodies. Each rustling blade is poking the next in excitement. The rain is coming! The hot summer days have exposed deep cracks in the dirt. The earth is opening her pores for some long-awaited moisture. I trace my finger along the crack as a beetle scurries for protection under a rounded stone and catch the first aroma of rain amidst the perfume of milkweed, yarrow, and sage blowing in the air. Everything has become quiet. The birds have silenced themselves; they have left their fluttering social communities and are now settled quietly into the clapping canopy of leaves above. I am aware of the increasing humidity on my skin as the sun begins to be covered, the sky becomes a shade of light brick red, and the rumbling grows louder. The only things still buzzing about are the mosquitos who are only now brave enough to come out with the sun behind the clouds. Although I cannot see it, I know that there is a small river here someplace—my uncle once shot a beaver from nearby his truck while I waited in the cab. He walked down the bank to retrieve it, and I remember covering my eyes as he tossed it into the box. A warm droplet of rain tickles my shoulder.

***

I returned in my memory to Manitoba as I prepared for this paper. It is something that I have continued to do in my studies—and for many reasons. Place is always the starting point for my research. This is the small place where my family's stories are from and from where I came. It is where our ancestors were born and where they died and where many have returned to the ground. Maria Campbell's recent keynote at the Mawachihitotaak Métis Studies Symposium only solidified my process. Over the online platform, she told the many Métis people gathered that "if we want to know who we are, you have to know your land, community, and your responsibilities to your people" (Campbell 2022). This resonated with us all. I know the land, people, and places that I come from. It is where our family has always been. The area that I come from in Manitoba spreads from Oakville to MacGregor, through Portage la Prairie, into Poplar Point, up Highway 26 into St Francois and Winnipeg and then into St. Andrews. This is the place where my Spence, Hallett, and Parenteau families married into the Fidler, Setter, Bird, Garrioch, and Foulds ones. Although I no longer live in this place, it still encompasses me: the smells, the sounds, and the tastes.

***

Today, I am on an overgrown remnant of a gravel road; today, I am not only observing my surroundings but also experiencing how the land, the birds, the insects, and the grasses interact and communicate within and between their societies, just as they always have. I am watching them shift their responses to a change in their environment.

But there is also a windrow of poplars here—the kind that someone always remembers being planted or to *have* planted in this place. On the left, I can just make out a small, tilted farmhouse that has become abandoned to the brush over time—its windows shot out years earlier, the wooden boards gnarled and burnt by the sun. Peonies and many lilac bushes still poking through the tall grass. Did you know that rows of planted lilacs often indicate where outhouses used to be? The roof is broken open. I recall being told that old so-and-so used to live in this place and that back in the day, this physical home used to be quite the place. There used to be some real parties there before the Second World War.

In the early 1920s and 1930s, my paternal great-great-grandparents Ernest Riggs and Mary Ann Spence's family would get together for a real rip-up. Uncle Stan would play his mother-of-pearl fiddle and tell the story about how one time, Uncle Totes (or, Ira Tryhurn, son of Frank Tryhurn and Emily

Foulds) and a woman were dancing—both, he would say, were a little on the heavy side. "Well wouldn't 'cha know,'" he would laugh, "they were dancing so hard they broke the cellar door and both fell three feet into the cellar." He had to stop playing and them found some boards, did a quick repair job, and promptly picked up the fiddle to get the party going again—everyone started dancing once more. When he told the story, he would laugh until he had tears in his eyes. My great-grandma Elsie, his sister, also loved a good laugh. She would let her imagination run wild and would laugh until she cried too. They danced the seven-step, three-step, Schottische, and heel-toe. The men drank and played cards or horseshoes while the women talked about making shirts and dresses with patterned flour bags. My Auntie Myrna says Great-Great-Auntie Elva, aka "just Auntie," would read tea leaves. She and her cousins would excitedly bring their tea leaves to learn their futures. Auntie would tell the girls that one of them would meet a guy and would describe what he looked like: "Like a rat," she would joke, "he has a long thin nose." The girls would laugh at their cousin's misfortune. Uncle Stan would surely have drunk too much by then and would sing "Darling We Are Growing Old, Silver Threads Among the Gold" to his wife, Laura Scofield, aka Dolly, and everyone would reminisce. Uncle Ray would bring along his tattoo gun and his recipes for making paint that he picked up in the First World War, and everyone would tell their stories about their lives on the prairies while teasing their brother that his upcoming marriage meant "releasing his other five prisoners."

***

To begin our conversations through the engagement with memories of who we are and where we come from is important. These memories are on the periphery of our own specific "homes," where our ancestors have lived for many generations. Our stories tie us to places and people that in turn tie us all together. Daniel Heath Justice (2016) writes that centering our experiences in our own stories is important (p. 26) because when we tell our stories, we are saying where and from whom we come. Stories are the foundation of our pasts, presents, and futures, and we are connected not only to each other but also to the land, our communities, our histories, and our ancestors in a multitude of ways. Through the (re)telling of our stories, we are enacting our relational obligation of *wahkohtowin* (Stevenson, 2021). Stories are our relations, and our identities and belonging are found within them. Flaminio et al. (2020) claim that visiting, both with the land and with our Métis relatives, has always been a "method of survival, of dialogue and deliberation, of decision-making, of responsibility, of celebration, and of sharing and caring for our relatives" (p. 55). Furthermore, when we continue to tell our stories, we are practicing our relational obligation to share our histories. Stories are our relations. Maria Campbell (2022) states during her keynote that stories are our kin and have their own power and agency. When we tell our stories, we say where and who we come from. To begin our research in this way is decolonizing and demonstrates Indigenous methodologies in action. And these memories, regardless of their outcomes, are authentic Indigenous experiences that speak to our histories, complexities, and diversity. These everyday stories have continued to shape who we are today.

Through many conversations with other Métis community members, scholars, and youth, it has become evident that several issues arise when speaking about how we fit into today's world as Métis people. We clearly cannot be the people that we read about in the pages of Canadian history and should not work to maintain a historic identity that is no longer in any way possible. As contemporary people, we must consider the effects of colonialism on our everyday realities, the passing of time, and our ancestors' agency to make decisions that would affect future generations. These factors have created many complexities and nuances that have resulted in our rich diversity. Yet many of us continue to look for ways to (re)connect. Many of us are looking for our way back to our communities, and I argue that this needs to begin with revisiting the land, the people, and the stories of where we are from. It is through the collection of these stories that we can see the intricacies of our histories and better understand our contemporary belonging to the Métis nation. It is through these stories of our everyday lives that we are witnessing the experiences of Métis people in real time.

Métis knowledge has always been connected to territory, kinship, and identity. These factors have remained intrinsic to how we understand the world. But in our busy lives, we sometimes forget to revisit the specific places we are from and the stories and memories that have been left within them. Furthermore, we must take the time to sit at the kitchen table and gather the day-to-day realities of how our communities *continue* to live and navigate the world as Indigenous people. I realize that these stories may not be as exciting as those that surround traditional or seemingly more authentic experiences. And yes, I understand that many of us want the excitement of the big stories of the past (I mean, we are Métis after all). But, over so many conversations with Métis people, I have recognized that many of us tend to center our belonging in notable historic Métis events and prominent names of the past. We continue to place ourselves in the context of "historic homelands" and names on scrip records. Of course, we want to know who your people are and where you are from. This is vital, even foundational. But to place our contemporary bodies into this past only continues to negate our present-day realities, denies our families' agency, and silences the multiplicities of our families' experiences. To leave ourselves in the past means not getting into the messiness of our identity struggles and our detachment from land, community, and language. We do not learn the reasons for silencing, protecting, and surviving. Our families have continued to navigate their specific locales and interact with the ever-changing political, economic, and social realities at specific times. We were not able to interact with our environment in the same ways that we were once accustomed to. Colonialism and settler society drew the parameters of what was important for society, and although they may have been of little value to us (and often further marginalizing), we were ultimately still forced to participate. This has created boundless diversity in who we are today. and yet many do not talk about these contemporary struggles.

Our experiences have both drawn us closer and pushed us farther from our communities. Over just a few generations, we have been forced to adapt to changes both inside and outside our control, and these adjustments were made in response to specific pressures that occurred in specific places at specific times. We must therefore balance each of our actions and experiences with the specific material lives, institutions, and processes that have influenced our local communities (Gregory, 1999). If we continue to narrow the scope of Métis experience by privileging larger macro-historical narratives that, as many Indigenous studies scholars have pointed out, privileges the history of white people—more specifically, white men—and feed into our contemporary invisibility, we stand to ignore our remarkable diversity. I have uncovered that we have had too many complex experiences that largely contradict how we have been imagined. As I have continued to articulate, our responses to the pressures in our specific locations have resulted in different narratives and complex forms of belonging that do not always fit neatly within the boundaries of "traditional" or "authentic" experience. We have urbanized and pursued our intellectual aims. We have made unions with people both inside and outside Métis communities and have chased educational, employment, and economic opportunities. We are not and can no longer be the historical people that are written about in history books because we are no longer in the past. There are many trees in the forest: many shrubs, many flowers, and many grasses. Each of our relations has roots that spread tightly around a very specific area—they are never truly detached, and some roots are plump and thick while others are barely detectable. Some roots cling tightly to each other and bind together, while others change paths to avoid large rocks in the earth. Some stretch out to attach to other root systems while others are way over there, in the farthest reaches, in search of water, nutrients, or stability—so far that you don't even know where they came from, but they are there. One thing for certain is that all roots begin in a central place and then extend outward. We have all had very specific circumstances that have changed our course, yet we remain Métis at our foundation. We need to talk about these changing courses through storytelling; as we tell our stories, we begin to learn about the gradual effects of colonialism.

We need to return to the teachings of *kiyokewin*; we must return to visiting and telling our stories. Our stories disclose the relationships, interactions, teachings, and events that have shaped us in the places we come from. We have an obligation to this kin. I want to dig in the dirt. I want to uncover the messiness of our identity struggles, our detachment from land, community, and language. I want to know about silencing, protecting, and survival. I want to know how the lilac bushes and peonies that could have otherwise been swallowed up by the native prairie grasses still bloom at the farmhouse after 100 years. I want to know all our stories about how we got here because we are the authors of our *own* animate theories about the world. I strive for stories that link the past to the realities of today.

***

We meet in following several texts to decide where we should go. Auntie Em sits in the middle of a Chicken Chef with pursed lips, showing me over coffee how to make a muskrat mating call while demonstrating how she would line up her shot on the side of the riverbank. We laugh about the idea of a white guy with a big piece of kielbasa wrapped around his square head as a mascot on a football jersey and then bellyache about how terrible the Winnipeg Jets are doing this year. On the same visit, some hot family tea is spilled, and the conversation leads to experiences of racism in the Portage la Prairie area. The cold winters are brought up. This shift leads to outlining the issues that Auntie Em faced being a half-breed in 1940s–1960s Manitoba—the issues she faced being Métis with a white dad. Getting beat up on the way home from school in the summer months because the other Métis kids who lived in Mud Town thought she was rich, and the complete rejection that she, her mother, and siblings endured from her father's white family. Her mother was denied any involvement in the local school, although she fiercely demanded her children be permitted to attend and receive an education. She continued to order library books from Winnipeg to keep her children educated. Auntie Em speaks about the embarrassment of ever bringing her white friends over and the racist remarks that she endured from old boyfriends. She speaks of hardships on the farm, and we go back to the summer: "You plant alfalfa before wheat, then barley, then oats, and then a summer haul—bah, your farming was probably just going to 7-Eleven in the city," and we laugh. She was not wrong; I wasn't called "The Princess" in my family for nothing. She has one of those great laughs where her face lights up and her whole body shakes. She giggles and has to run because she's late for church . . . and of course offers to pay for *my* lunch.

***

We collectively bear a responsibility to share the diverse narratives that have shaped us and to address gaps in our understanding and memory. In so doing, we should not just recount stories that echo our past identities; instead, we should focus on sharing narratives that reflect the journeys to who we have become today.

References

Campbell, M. (2022). Respecting each other's bundles [Keynote presentation]. Mawachihitotaak Métis Studies Symposium, Winnipeg. Manitoba, Canada, May 6, 2022.

Flaminio, A. C., Gaudet, J. C., & Dorion, L. M. (2022). Métis women gathering: Visiting together and voicing wellness for ourselves. *AlterNative: An International Journal of Indigenous Peoples, 16*(1), 55–63. https://doi.org/10.1177/1177180120903499

Gaudet, J. C. (2019). Keeoukaywin: The visiting way—Fostering an Indigenous research methodology. *Aboriginal Policy Studies, 7*(2), 47–64. https://doi.org/10.5663/aps.v7i2.29336

Gregory, B. (1999). Is small beautiful? Microhistory and the history of everyday life. In *History and Theory, 38*(1), 100–110. https://doi.org/10.1111/0018-2656.791999079

Heath Justice, D. (2016) Reflections on Indigenous literary nationalism: On home grounds, singing hogs, and cranky critics. In C. Andersen and J. O'Brien (Eds.), *Sources and Methods in Indigenous Studies* (pp. 23–30). Routledge.

Stevenson, A. D. (2021). *Intimate integration: A history of the Sixties Scoop and the colonization of Indigenous*. University of Toronto Press.

· 13 ·

LEARNING TO LISTEN CLOSELY: THE LISTENING GUIDE AND "I POEMS" IN MÉTIS RESEARCH METHODOLOGIES

Lucy Delgado

Introduction and Positionality

In reflecting on the Mawachihitotaak Métis Studies Symposium, I am filled with gratitude for all the work that was done and the spaces created for Métis scholars, artists, and community members to come together and share some of their expertise. With this in mind, maarsii for taking the time to read my experiences with a relational data analysis method, the listening guide (LG).

But first—taanshi! Lucy Delgado d-ishinikaashon, Winnipeg d-oschin. En Michif niya. I am Lucy Delgado, a Métis two-spirit woman, born in Winnipeg to a Métis mother and a biological father of Irish descent. My ancestors on my mother's side took scrip in St. Andrews, Manitoba, after leaving homes farther north in York Factory, Oxford House, and Norway House. My settler ancestry comes from Carlow, Ireland, and the Orkney Islands. I am a community member, an educator, a sister, a daughter, a spouse, and a mother. All these facets of my being have come together in my research and the work that I do.

In this chapter, I discuss my doctoral research and the data analysis process that I used while conducting it. I also share what I know and am still learning about Métis research methodologies and the ways I think this method of analysis fits into methodologies that center Métis ontologies.

Framing the Research

The research study focused on the experiences of Métis youth who engage in hip-hop cultures. I undertook this work as an extension of my master's research, in which I had (unintentionally) only worked with Métis men, and I wanted to be sure to prioritize the inclusion of women and 2SLGBTQ+ people. To achieve this goal, I applied an additional lens of interrogation of the experiences of 2SLGBTQ+ (or queer) youth. My research aimed to uncover the experiences of queer Métis youth who engaged in hip-hop as producers or fans and to learn about their experiences with education.

I am a queer Métis person who has found solace and joy in hip-hop cultures, so this work was deeply connected to who I am. The doctoral research took place under exceptional circumstances; the first iteration of the research design was approved just weeks before the coronavirus pandemic hit, and the process had to be reimagined for a digital space. Over Zoom, I interviewed eight Métis young people, seven of whom were queer and all of whom had participated in hip-hop cultures—that is, rapping, graffiti, dance, spoken word, street style, and other aspects—at some point in their lives. These interviews were conversational, inspired by the visiting method and the concept of kiyokewin, which I discuss in the following section.

Métis Research Methodologies

Centering this research around a Métis-specific methodology was important to me in designing this project, but I held the words of LaVallee et al. (2016) as a reminder that "there is not one Métis identity, thus, not one Métis methodology" (p. 170). The methodology used in this study drew from Métis theorists like Gaudet (2019) and Flaminio et al. (2020) who wrote about visiting, or kiyokewin, as a research methodology that centers on relationality. Visiting, which typically happens in person with shared food and stories, is a way that Métis people strengthen their relationships and kinship ties and pass on knowledge (Flaminio et al., 2020; Gaudet, 2019). Given that this research design happened concurrently with the beginning of the COVID-19 pandemic, these spaces were conceived of digitally. While we could not share food, the participants and I shared laughter, stories, and pieces of ourselves.

Kiyokewin as a methodology is also closely linked to kitchen table methodologies as conceptualized by Black feminist scholars like Davis (1999), Smith (1989), and Bennett (2006), queer Mestiza/Latina feminist scholars like Delgado Bernal (2001), and Métis scholars both established (Mattes, 2016) and emerging (Ferland, 2022). This focus on spaces that are oriented toward community and relationality was integral to the project, and relationships were not limited to the data collection process and connections with participants. That approach also guided the way I entered into a relationship with the data themselves. In the LG (or voice-centered) relational approach to data analysis, I found a method that matched this attention to care, relationship, and reciprocity.

The LG and I Poems

The LG was first developed and used by Carol Gilligan in the field of psychology. Gilligan (1982) had noticed that in her field, the stories and experiences of men were treated as the benchmark for human behavior against which women's experiences were measured, and the literature overwhelmingly treated men's perspectives as neutral. Throughout the early 1990s, the LG method was developed and deployed by Gilligan and graduate students at Harvard University and has since been used in a wide variety of subject areas, including nursing, policing, health research, and education.

The series of successive listenings (or close readings) that comprise the LG method allow the researcher to bore more deeply into the data with each round. The first round of listening is for the plot, in order to identify what is happening in the story the participant is telling. Who are the characters? Where does the story take place? What is happening? This listening is also an opportunity for researchers to acknowledge their reactions to the plot, write down any thoughts that arise, or note any memories that come back. With these reactions, researchers make clear the connections between what is happening in the data and their own experiences.

The next listening is for the "I" voice. In this round, researchers return to the beginning of the data and pull out any statements that begin with "I" (or sometimes "I" and "we"), including the verb and, sometimes, the object of the clause. These are moved to another document that begins to take the shape of what Gilligan et al. (2003) call "I poems." These poems are meant to give a glimpse into the participant's subconscious and reveal patterns of thought.

The third listening, which can be comprised of multiple listenings, is for contrapuntal voices. That term is borrowed from music theory and refers to the idea that listeners can attune their ears to different instruments, harmonies, or dissonances (Mauthner, 2017). After this step, the researchers can look at the data and think about them within the broader context of the research. Does what emerged from these listenings address the research questions? Is there another lens that could be applied to get closer to the root of the research problem? In this work, I completed several additional listenings to focus on where learning happens for the participants and how that happens.

As a method, the LG is deeply rigorous and time-consuming, but the way that researchers become entrenched in the data is nothing short of remarkable (Chu, 2004). With each successive reading, I felt that I knew the participants more deeply. Through acknowledging and writing down my own reactions, I was able to have a conversation with the data and with my own subconscious. I now focus on several of the I poems that emerged from these data. I share snippets of those poems, as each participant's stories created pages and pages of I poems to consider.

The I Poems

As noted above, the second listening of the data is to create I poems by pulling out any first-person statements and contextual language and placing these sentences in a document, each on a new line. While transcribing the I poems, I found myself falling into the routine of copying and pasting from one document to the next without a sharp focus on the words or meaning behind them. Once the I poems had been collated, I decided to return to them and divide them into stanzas corresponding both to the transcripts and the rhythms of what was being said. Reading through these sentences again shifted my view of the words from disjointed phrases to the poetry they were meant to be.

One participant, Marcus, met with me twice. In our first conversation, Marcus told me that he didn't know if he should use the term two-spirit or where he fit in as a Métis man who was just learning about his own sexuality. The topic of two-spirit identity came up again in our second conversation. Part of the I poem from our second conversation read:

> I struggle with
> I've had a lot of struggle with
> I know there are two-spirit people
> I guess wounds and trauma that are all around
> I don't know anywhere you can go
> I mean

This stanza of the poem ends with the words hanging in the air, a palpable representation of Marcus's uncertainty. He has struggled with his own identity and how that identity fits into community and even what supports are available to him. However, a few stanzas later, Marcus shifts the topic to his children and their identities, and the tone changes as well.

> I – I'm cool with the fluidity
> I don't push it on him
> I call him a boy
> I call him kid
> (Have I called him a girl?)
> I tell him
> I like his dresses and stuff
> I just—I just let him be
> I wouldn't say—I wouldn't say no
> I wouldn't shoot him down
> I would let him play
> I don't think I'm ready to

Marcus's child has shown interest in being fluid with his gender expression by wearing dresses, which Marcus has supported. While Marcus tells us that he would not try to force his child into one gender role, he also reflects on whether he is demonstrating neutrality. He asks himself aloud if he has ever called his child a girl or if he has only used the terms "boy" and "kid." Marcus is happy to let his child be who they are and would support any gender identity they claimed, but he does not "think [he's] ready to" give himself that space to explore or "play" with his own gender identity.

The I poem of another participant, Kenna, also touched on being uncomfortable exploring her queer identity. When speaking about a group of her friends, she said the following:

> I noticed that
> I know they're not okay with gay people
> I don't agree with that, obviously
> I think that that's stupid
> I still like them as people
> if I came out
> I don't know
> I know that if I come out, they're not going to dump me as friends
> I'm not sure I'm ready to deal
> I think they would be scared of me
> I'm not really ready for that
> I'm just

> I have to deal with them so much
> I don't really want to have that experience
> I think that it would—it would be weird

This group of friends is one with whom Kenna hasn't felt comfortable sharing her queer identity. She tells us that she doesn't think the friendships would end if she came out, but they "would be scared" of her, and it would be a "weird" experience, one she is not ready for. Part of the LG method involves bringing the researcher's experiences to the forefront, and this I poem brought me back to my own stories. In my doctoral dissertation (Fowler, 2022), I wrote about experiencing bullying in elementary school for my sexuality. From that, I learned how to perform heterosexuality and conform to a specific type of gender presentation to avoid being targeted. I hid parts of my identity from friends, family, and partners for many years and only recently began to assert myself in queer spaces. I wonder whether—had I been interviewed at Kenna's age—I would have shared similar stories and what I might say to a younger me.

Conclusion

These I poem excerpts demonstrate the importance of listening carefully to not only the words spoken by participants but the pauses and patterns in how they talk about themselves. The LG approach holds that the words we choose often reveal underlying feelings or thoughts that we might not even be aware of. This method has been used to analyze interviews, historical documents, and even quantitative data—I look forward to continuing to use it and learn other ways it can be deployed in my research journey.

The I poems and the LG more generally also encourage the researcher to engage in self-reflection and to see themselves and their experiences in the words of the participants. In this way, the LG method connects deeply to research done in a Métis framework centered on Métis ontologies and honors relationships—between researchers and participants, researchers and data, and researchers and themselves.

References

Bennett, K. (2006). Kitchen drama: Performances, patriarchy and power dynamics in a Dorset. *Gender, Place and Culture: A Journal of Feminist Geography, 13*(2), 153–160. https://doi.org/10.1080/09663690600573775

Chu, Judy Y. (2004). A relational perspective on adolescent boys' identity development. In N. Chu & Judy Y. Way (Eds.), *Adolescent boys: Exploring diverse cultures of boyhood* (pp. 78–105). New York University Press.

Davis, O. I. (1999). In the kitchen: Transforming the academy through safe spaces of resistance. *Western Journal of Communication*, 63(3), 364–381. https://doi.org/10.1080/10570319909374647

Delgado Bernal, D. (2001). Learning and living pedagogies of the home: The Mestiza consciousness of Chicana students. *International Journal of Qualitative Studies in Education*, 14(5), 623–639. https://doi.org/10.1080/09518390110059838

Ferland, N. (2022). *"We're still here": Teaching and learning about Métis women's and two-spirit people's relationships with land in Winnipeg* [Master's thesis, University of Saskatchewan]. https://hdl.handle.net/10388/13931

Flaminio, A. G., Gaudet, J. C., & Dorion, L. M. (2020). Métis women gathering: Visiting together and voicing wellness for ourselves. *AlterNative: An International Journal of Indigenous Peoples*, 16(1): 55–63. https://doi.org/10.1177/1177180120903499. https://doi.org/10.1177/1177180120903499.

Fowler, Lucy. (2017). *We're rapping not trapping: Hip hop as a contemporary expression of Métis culture and a conduit to literacy* [Master's thesis, Lakehead University]. https://knowledgecommons.lakeheadu.ca/handle/2453/4169

Fowler, Lucy. (2022). *Where learning happens: Conversations with queer, Métis youth who engage in hip-hop cultures* [Doctoral dissertation, University of Saskatchewan]. https://harvest.usask.ca/handle/10388/13941

Gaudet, J. C. (2019). Keeoukaywin: The visiting way: Fostering an Indigenous research methodology. *Aboriginal Policy Studies*, 7(2), pp. 47–64. https://doi.org/10.5663/aps.v7i2.29336

Gilligan, C. (1982). *In a different voice: Psychological theory and women's development*. Harvard University Press.

Gilligan, C., & Eddy, J. (2017). Listening as a path to psychological discovery: An introduction to the listening guide. *Perspectives in Medical Education*, 6, 76–81. https://doi.org/10.1007/s40037-017-0335-3

Gilligan, C, Spencer, R., Weinberg, M. K., & Bertsch, T. (2003). On the listening guide: A voice-centered relational method. In P. M. Camie, J. E. Rhodes, & L. Yardley (Eds.), *Qualitative research in psychology: Expanding perspectives in methodology and design* (p. 157–172). American Psychological Association.

LaVallee, A., Troupe, T., & Turner, T. (2016). Negotiating and exploring relationships in Métis community-based research. *Engaged Scholar Journal: Community-Engaged Research, Teaching and Learning*, 2(1), 167–182. https://esj.usask.ca/index.php/esj/article/view/61485/46494

Mattes, C. (2012). *Curating as kitchen table talk* [Video]. Plug In Institute of Contemporary Art, 2012. https://vimeo.com/177302420

Mauthner, N. S. (2017). The listening guide feminist method of narrative analysis: Towards a posthumanist performative (re)configuration. In J. Woodiwiss, K. Smith, & K. Lockwood (Eds.), *Feminist narrative research* (pp. 65–91). Palgrave Macmillan

Smith, B. (1989). A press of our own kitchen table: Women of color press. *Frontiers (Boulder)*, 10(3), 11–13. https://doi.org/10.2307/3346433

· 14 ·

I COULD TURN INTO A RIVER WHEN I WAS A GIRL: CROOKED METHODOLOGIES AND THE GATHERING RESEARCH FRAMEWORK

Michelle Porter

Introduction

When I am invited to read from my creative work, I sometimes begin by sharing with the listeners that I could turn into a river when I was a girl. I tell my audience how much I miss being a river and that it's a lot harder to do now with the beginnings of arthritis and stiff joints. I say, "rivers are my relations and all my life they've offered different stories about belonging." In doing this, my intention is to invoke my kinship with rivers and offer an informal introduction to two aspects of my approach to research and writing: crookedness and gatherings.

Crooked methodology is a Métis-specific approach to research-creation that has been part of my practice since my first postdoctoral fellowship in 2019. The notion of gathering describes the relationship between academic research and creativity in my work. By introducing crooked methodologies and home-as-gathering, I offer insights into the practical and theoretical frameworks through which relational Métis research and/or research-creation can be practiced. From a *fiddling point of view* (the relevance and context of which are discussed below), I am sharing how I play my song and say, "Now that you've heard this song, you can play it in your own way and make it yours."

Who I Am

I am a descendant of the Goulet family from the Red River settlements established in the late 1700s in Manitoba. My great-grandfather, a fiddle performer named Robert Leon Goulet, made some of the earliest recordings of Métis music. He gave up on the promise of the scrip land and moved with his family to British Columbia. My grandmother's and mother's generations became part of the Métis diaspora, many of whom moved again and again in search of a place to build a home. Hence, mobility-as-resilience and mobility-as-survival among some of Canada's Métis people have been the subject of my most recent research and writing.

After listening so many times to recordings of my ancestors' music, including some recorded at the home of my grandmother and great-grandfather, I have come to understand myself as a descendant of a long line of Métis storytellers who used music to share their stories. I have been deeply conscious of the fact that I tell my stories using words and not the fiddle. I am a scholar and creative writing professor and have published a number of books, including a book of poetry titled *Inquiries* (2019), two creative nonfiction books, *Approaching Fire* (2020) and *Scratching River* (2022b), and one novel, *A Grandmother Begins the Story* (2023). During the processes of researching and writing these books, I worked within the crooked and gathering frameworks outlined in this chapter.

Research-Creation

Indigenous arts practices and knowledge systems are embedded in the imagination, and creation of possible futures are central to Indigenous continuity (Lewis, 2017). Research-creation involves arts practices that "matter not only in the sense of being relevant to the world but in the actual material of this and future worlds as well" (Washuta & Warburton, 2019, p. 15). Drawing on Stévance and Lacasse (2013), I see that research-creation can be a circular process in which research and creation work together to produce fuller understandings than either could produce on its own, but I also see the possibility of research-creation taking other shapes. It could be a tool for interrogating and interrupting common assumptions about research, such as the principle data gathering must be followed by research dissemination. In the work I do, research-creation is a tool that imaginatively connects data with story. The frameworks in this paper termed crooked and gathering are two shapes or movements in which the research-creation process can bring life to data and art. These approaches reach across time, often in a non-linear fashion, and for this reason can be a tool not only of reconciliation but also of future creation.

Crooked Methodologies

The tradition of Métis fiddle and dance tunes inspired my approach to research. Specifically, I applied the term *crooked* to some of my research-creation work. The Métis music and dance traditions I refer to arose from a convergence of First Nations and European traditions. The Métis embraced these traditions and made them their own. *Crookedness* refers to the way Métis fiddlers add or drop a beat or change the rhythm according to their particular artistic expression in varying phrase lengths and asymmetric structures. It is that crookedness that I have brought to my interdisciplinary academic journey.

I want to make clear that I am neither a dancer nor a fiddler. I am a writer looking to her ancestors' music and dance traditions for direction and inspiration in storytelling—I am listening carefully to these traditions. When jigging certain dances, such as the Red River Jig, dancers listen to the music for signal to move from traditional dance steps to fancy steps (often called "the change"), which take the form of new steps or contemporary dance steps. In this, fiddle playing and jigging are *gatherings* that pull from the past and the present, making room for future dance steps and for the next generation's interpretations of the dance. To make this happen, however, dancers have to listen carefully:

> Most Métis fiddlers learned to play by ear and didn't read music. They began adding extra beats which is why it is now known as "crooked" music.[1]
>
> Everyone plays it a little differently so you [the dancers] really have to listen carefully for the changes in the music or you'll be offbeat.[2]

Following in those dance steps, research-creation uses art to engage the circularity of the present, past, and future, making space for "telling Métis stories and generating the real-world empowerment of Métis communities" (Gaudry, 2021, p. 220). Research-creation can thus engage with a wide range of complex ideas about Métis music, dance, culture, and identity—and what will become of them in the future. This kind of imaginative approach is a vital first step toward decolonizing our conception of our present, past, and future relationships. The crucial role of art was recognized over a century ago when Louis Riel wrote, "My people will sleep for one hundred years but when they awake, it will be the artists who give them their spirit back." In my own words, research-creation is the process of taking different kinds of knowledge and playing them like a song by a traditional Métis fiddler or as if I were dancing along with a traditional jig, just like my great-grandfather, Bob Goulet.

Gatherings

Elsewhere, I have argued that geographies of home/land(s) can be understood through a "gathering framework" (Porter, 2016) that makes room for the many and varied relational networks and mobilities through which we reach our home/land(s). Broadly, this approach is a Métis-centered response to capitalist, Eurocentric notions of home and claims to home. Because the creation of art is one of the many gatherings through which home and land are created, claimed, and sustained, in this section I discuss the relationship between research-creation and gatherings.

The introduction to *Indigenous Poetics* (McLeod, 2014) suggests that Indigenous artists move beyond writing about dislocation and write instead about remaking home. Lewis (2017) developed an interactive research-creation project that does just that, providing imaginative future-based spaces for Indigenous youth in digital arenas, including video game narratives. He wrote about the relevance of "the question of how Indigenous people imagine our future, and the related questions of how we will build our way to that future" (Lewis, 2017, para. 2). If research-creation can be part of building a future home (as Métis people and communities, as families, as individuals), then we can better understand those imaginative, arts-based home geographies of the future using the notion of gathering.

The verb *gather* can mean "bring or come together, assemble, accumulate; infer or deduce; summon up (energy, etc.); pick or collect as harvest; increase (speed); draw together in folds or wrinkles; develop purulent swelling" (*The Oxford Dictionary of Current English*) or more broadly

> to bring together and take in from scattered places or sources; to pick up from the ground or a surface; collect (grain or crops) as a harvest (or plants, fruits etc. for food); draw together or toward oneself, as in "she gathered the child in her arms"; draw and hold together (fabric or a part of a garment) by running thread through it; infer or understand; summon up a mental or physical attribute (such as one's thoughts or one's strength) for a purpose. (*The New Oxford American Dictionary*)

These various definitions unravel a concept that is deeply embedded with movement. Seen this way, gatherings are always beginning and ending and reconstituting themselves in response to changes in time, people, material and physical surroundings, and imaginations. If we look for connections between home and ways of gathering, we can see the coming and going of connections and/or relations that constitute the meaning and physical reality of home.

In the research-creation process, gatherings are drawn from a wide range of materials (e.g., words, dance steps, musical instruments, paint, beads) in order to create particular relationships with the past, the present, and a desired future. Every work of art is made up of its own gatherings. In this chapter I focus on the ways that notions of gathering and crookedness have shaped my own work.

Praxis: Using Gatherings and Crookedness in Arts Creation

Each of my books is a gathering, a process in which I was trying to create, recreate, or sustain connections to home and land across time. My first nonfiction exploration of these gatherings became *Approaching Fire* (2020), which is related to the form of crooked music by straying from many of the standard expectations and rhythms of nonfiction prose. The book moves between genres and refuses to grant the consistency often asked of standard nonfiction works. There are unexpected improvisations and dropped notes and added phrases throughout the book. *Approaching Fire* is also connected to Brenda Macdougall's work on the social landscape of Métis communities, but that connection is not made in a straight line. Rather, this story of a social landscape unfolds in my book through a mix of poetry, prose, letters, and newspaper clippings from the 1930s. *Approaching Fire* is important for me personally because it focuses on the family unit that made up my grandfather's band, the Red River Echoes. Leanne Simpson (2014) suggests that "our ancestors often acted within the family unit to physically survive, to pass on what they could to their children" (p. 16). In the book, I tell the story of my discovery of my great-grandfather's and grandmother's music. I weave theoretical discussions into narratives of my grandfather's and grandmother's personal experiences with music.

In the process of gathering all these research elements together, I discovered for myself an important relational tool. Working through early drafts, I was struck by how the book was *about* my great-grandfather, a man I didn't know except through stories. I began searching for ways to build a relationship with him. Near the end of the writing process, I began writing letters to him that formed the melody of the book and made it about my relationship with my grandfather. By the end, I came to develop a real relationship with him, even though I had never met him. By allowing the gathering of all these elements on the page, I changed my real-life connection to an ancestor I had not known in person. In so doing, I also built a future in which I could learn from him.

Scratching River (2022b) is a collection of stories and voices braided on the page to create order from the sometimes chaotic rhythm of actual lived experience and memory. I use oral histories, stories, maps, personal autobiography, and historical documents as sources. Scratching River foregrounds the story of a search for a home for my older brother, who has dual diagnoses of schizophrenia and autism.

I wrote Scratching River to better understand my own place in the Métis nation and my own historical relationship to mobility and home. That my brother's story appeared as a result of this arts-based research process was entirely unexpected. And yet, there he is, at the center of it all. It was this process of consciously gathering elements, including rivers, roads, travel, homeland, ancestor, sister, mother, mental illness, and self that I changed how I understood the violence that had happened to my brother. The gathering that is this book led to a healing that changed how I understand key points of my family's past and where we are going, of our future. In writing this book I came to a better understanding of my brother's own journey.

There's also a crookedness in Scratching River, a dropped note in the form of refusal. Its fragmented and braided structure is the refusal to fill in the gaps left by violence, the refusal to provide the reader with an easy, satisfying closure, and the refusal to reinstate into the text the violence that structures a complex family and home history. Through these refusals, my book became a critical re-reading of one Métis family's place in geography, time, and circumstance. My book evolves into an embodied reading of the land and intergenerational knowledge and connections.

Following the Bison: Another Kind of Crooked Approach

In my newest work, bison have joined the gatherings that bring together an ecosystem-based research-creation project. By focusing on Métis relationships with bison, I explored and am still exploring in fiction what it meant to be Métis in the past, what being Métis means today, and what it could mean in the future. This involves the braiding of science, traditional ecological knowledge, oral history, arts and creativity, and, of course, stories.

The bison, or the *bufloo* in Michif, the Métis language, was not only a keystone grassland species, but was the "great shaggy guardian of the western doorway, stands within the realm of reason"; the bison originally taught the Métis how to live life through a process of "mutual exchange between all beings, individuals and groups" (Leclair, 2003, p. 62).

Today, bison can teach us about survival and returning to land-based relationships. In recent years we have been witnessing a number of efforts to facilitate the return of bison to the prairies and to restore grasslands across Canadian Prairies and the United States Great Plains. Bison can help us build a future where they will continue to live in kinship with us here on the prairies, but we don't yet have enough stories to lead the way. This bison-centered project explores Jennifer Adese's (2014) call for "understandings of Métis kinship that neither begin nor end with inter-human relations" and stories that "ensure the continuance of Métis world views, expose the impact of colonial processes on Métis and call us [Métis] home to remember our relationships to our ecosystems" (pp. 50–51).

It was from these beginnings that I wrote my first novel, *A Grandmother Begins the Story*. My novel uses different sets of gatherings through the telling of stories from both bison and human perspectives in an examination of the power of memory to repair our relationships with ourselves, our families, the land we belong to, and the future we want to create.

Toward a Conclusion

In this chapter I have introduced the methodological and theoretical concepts of crookedness and gathering that have become central to my research and writing practices. I do this in the spirit of my great-grandfather, who would share his songs with other fiddlers so that they could take his music and make it their own if it spoke to them. In academic language, I am sharing key practical and theoretical frameworks that can guide relational Métis research and/or research-creation. I often end public readings with the final poem of my poetry book, *Inquiries*, and I do so here to honor the role rivers have played in my life, in my ancestors' lives, and in my research and writing.

Childhood, Remembered

as a girl
she could turn into a river.
when she wanted to get away from here
and go there, she only had to lay down
and lean into the easiest route.
the going and arriving happened all at once—
she was always tumbling down rocks and cliffs
beneath the slant of the sun at the same time as she
pooled, still as a mountain, at the place she never, ever
finished going to.

Notes

1 thedancecentre.ca/story/yvonne-chartrand-on-metis-dances/ (accessed March 11, 2024).
2 www.vnidansi.ca/company/interview-yvonne-about-red-river-jig (accessed March 11, 2024).

References

Gaudry, A. (2011). Insurgent research. *Wicazo Sa Review*, 26(1), 113–136.
Gaudry, A. (2018). Communing with the dead: The "new Métis," Métis identity appropriation, and the displacement of living Métis culture. *American Indian Quarterly*, 42(2), 162–190. https://www.jstor.org/stable/10.5250/amerindiquar.42.2.0162
Gaudry, A. (2021). Building the field of Métis studies: Toward transformative and empowering Métis scholarship. In J. Adese & C. Andersen (Eds.), *A people and a nation: New directions in contemporary Métis studies* (pp. 213–229). UBC Press.
Justice, D. H. (2018). *Why Indigenous literatures matter*. WLU Press.
Leclair, C. (1998). Métis wisdom: Learning and teaching across the cultures. *Atlantis*, 22(2), 123–126. https://journals.msvu.ca/index.php/atlantis/article/view/3454
Leclair, C. (2002). Memory alive: Race, religion and Métis identities. *Essays on Canadian Writing*, 75(7), 126–144.
Leclair, C. (2003). *Métis environmentalism: La tayr pi tout li moond* [Unpublished doctoral dissertation]. York University.
Lewis, J. E. (2016), A brief (media) history of the Indigenous future. *PUBLIC: Art, Culture, Ideas*, 54(4), 36–49.
Lewis, J. E. (2017). About. *Initiative for Indigenous Futures, Aboriginal Territories in Cyberspace*. Retrieved November 11, 2022, from https://indigenousfutures.net/about/
McLeod, N. (2014). *Indigenous poetics in Canada*. WLU Press.

Porter, M. (2016). *Moving home: Narrating place, home, and rurality in Newfoundland and Labrador* [Doctoral dissertation, Memorial University of Newfoundland]. https://research.library.mun.ca/12422/

Porter, M. (2019). *Inquiries*. Breakwater Books.

Porter, M. (2020). *Approaching fire*. Breakwater Books.

Porter, M. (2022a, May 3–6). *Crooked methodologies: Working between arts-based research, bison-centred knowledge* [Paper presentation]. Mawachihitotaak Métis Studies Symposium, Winnipeg, MB, Canada.

Porter, M. (2022b). *Scratching river*. WLU Press.

Porter, M. (2023). *A grandmother begins the story*. Penguin.

Stévance, S., & Lacasse, S. (2022). *Research-creation in music and the arts: Towards a collaborative interdiscipline*. Taylor & Francis Group.

Washuta, E., & Warburton, T. (2019). Introduction. In E. Washuta & T. Warburton (Eds.), *Shapes of Native nonfiction: Collected essays by contemporary writers* (pp. 3–20). University of Washington Press.

· 15 ·

STORYING MÉTIS SEXUALITIES: MÉTIS CONFESSIONS: OUR FIRST TIME—RED RIVER EDITION

Angie Tucker, KD King (Sangria Jiggz), Tanya Ball and Paul L. Gareau

Content Warning

This essay contains colonially imposed illicit mature content including open conversations about sex and sexuality, rape, and suggestive language. We reject narratives of violence that have historically surrounded Indigenous sexuality, stand with those who have been victims of sexual abuse, and see this work as a site of resurgence to resist the colonial repression of our sexual diversity and the plurality of our gender roles and sexual practices.

> I confess … sometimes when I'm home alone or after the kids have gone to bed, I'll put on anything with Jeff Goldblum, even *Jurassic Park*; there's something about his voice, and I lay under a blanket and listen to his voice with my eyes closed. It makes me so wet. (Anonymous confession, 2022)

We confess that this essay will be much like our actual first time. Yes! The thought of curling up with us in a sweaty bundle of HBC wool blankets and silky furs is exciting. But before you get your hopes up, we must warn you that we end quickly and a bit sloppily. But—as in all things—practice makes perfect. Our practice comes through Métis Confessions, a cousin of Tipi Confessions, a storytelling event that celebrates, respects, and connects Indigenous peoples to our kinship responsibility of being in good relations with all genders and sexualities. Tipi Confessions was founded in 2015 by Kim TallBear, Savage Bear, and Kirsten Lindquist as an offshoot of "Bedpost Confessions," a storytelling show originating in Austin, Texas. Tipi Confessions uses a decolonizing lens to provide curated stories and performances that expose the vulnerability, humor, confusion, and sexy details of Indigenous sex and sexuality.

The Foreplay

Angie: My name is Angie Tucker (she/her), and I am a PhD student in the Faculty of Native Studies at the University of Alberta. I am a Métis mother, wife, sister, daughter, auntie, and friend who grew up in Winnipeg, Manitoba. My family stories begin in St. Andrews and in the Poplar Point–Portage la Prairie area of Manitoba, and I have deep connections to these spaces and my relationships in them. As co-thinkers of the first Mawachihitotaak Métis Studies Symposium, Paul L. Gareau and I were passionate about volunteering for any role that was available. We recognized the powerful impact that this event would have on Métis youth, community members, Elders, and scholars—and for me, the land at Red River was calling me home. As luck (and clear obviousness if you have met either of us) would have it, we both found ourselves on the social committee. After almost two years of living with the COVID-19 pandemic, the social committee was optimistic that we would be able to gather for any number of important events, and Paul and I kept thinking, "What do we do with everyone who is visiting and looking for things to do in the evenings?" This question caused Paul and I to branch into a separate division of the social committee that was dubbed the "Métis After Dark" team. Paul and I loved it! Our minds raced with potential events such as Indigenous karaoke, Indigenous drag shows, a dinner at a locally owned Métis restaurant, or a name-that-tune pub night at a local Indigenous venue, but none of these stacked up against our ultimate goal. We wanted something truly unforgettable. We wanted to ask if Tipi Confessions would be willing to travel to Winnipeg to host a Métis-specific event. We contacted Kim TallBear, Kirsten Lindquist, and Savage Bear and were sad to learn that they did not have the capacity to pull a show together at that time. But we were honored (and terrified) when they suggested that we host an event on our own. We titled the event Métis Confessions: Our First Time—Red River Edition.

The thought of the "first time" brought forward past trauma. In contemplation of taking over the role of host, I questioned whether I would even be physically, emotionally, mentally, or spiritually able to contribute to this project. Although I have always been open to talking about sex and sexuality, I have also experienced deep discomfort in confronting the ways that non-consensual sex has affected my life. I have not been able to adequately explain how it has continued to traumatize me well into my adult years, nor am I able to fully articulate how assault goes far beyond the act itself—beyond the relationship that you have with your body and beyond the distorted views about giving and receiving pleasure. It is because of sex that I have had to work through negative feelings about myself. It is because of sex that I have struggled with trust, the need for control, the fear of being abandoned, and feeling unsafe. It is because of sex that I continue to question people's motives. And it is because of sex that I struggle with anxiety and worry about how others perceive me. It is because of sex that I looked for ways to alter my thoughts through drugs and alcohol in my youth. When your body is taken, manipulated, and exploited, it responds in any number of unexpected ways. Like the land once it is exploited, our bodies never return to us in their original state:

> Native women's bodies were to the settler eye, like land, therefore the Native woman is "unrapeable" (or "highly rapeable") because she was like land, matter to be extracted from, used, sullied, taken from, over and over again, something that is already violated and violatable. (Simpson, 2017, p. 6)

We know that Indigenous women have continued to play significant cultural, spiritual, and political roles in our communities and that it is through our mothers, aunties, and sisters that we learn about sex and sexuality, gender, and intimacy through storytelling, ceremonies, and songs. Sometimes the information that is relayed surrounds love, childbearing, emotional connection, our relations with non-human entities, and the exploration of our own bodies. However, other aspects surround the deeper issues of being violated and assaulted. Clearly, some of us choose not to talk about these more serious issues. We lock away our feelings of shame and self-blame and never adequately deal with the repercussions of having our bodies and minds abused by those we trusted. Many of us look for ways to suppress our negative experiences without confronting how we have been shaped by them. But as I have learned over time, we must separate our negative sexual experiences from those that are healthy and positive. Although we must honor our resilience to have worked so hard to protect our spirits and minds from the hurtful assaults we have endured, it is possible to learn to trust and to put ourselves in the vulnerable position of consensually sharing our bodies with those who love and respect us. Through storytelling, it is the women in our families who have taught us how to protect ourselves and work through our pain, grief, and fears. And through these types of conversations, we uncover the gendered legacy of colonialism and the historical and political systems of oppression that have continued to provide spaces for these acts of violence to continue to occur.

Sarah Deer confronts the effects of colonial oppression on Indigenous women's bodies and strives to locate intersectional approaches that can assist in the eradication of endemic sexual violence and abuse in tribal communities. In order to heal as sovereign Indigenous peoples, Deer (2015) insists that we must "look to our histories, beliefs, resources, and experiences to reclaim the safety and empowerment for all women" (p. 122). With this statement, I am reminded of the obligations that we have to our community. I recognized that one of the ways that I can help to protect and empower other Indigenous women (and men and non-gender-conforming people) is not by silencing my discomfort with talking about the complexities of sex. We must focus on supporting and strengthening the collective health, safety, and wellbeing of our people and stress the positive aspects of Indigenous sex and sexuality.

In addition to Deer's work, I have been empowered by Dian Million's (2009) felt theory to think about the ways that I can speak openly about my experiences while embracing and sharing my emotional knowledge. As I contemplated my ability to contribute to this production, I recognized that as an Indigenous feminist scholar who aims to deconstruct the racialized and gendered nature of colonization, I must directly engage with the repercussions that colonization has had on our sexual bodies. The abuse and victimization of our bodies can no longer be silenced or rendered invisible, and it is through felt conversation that we can work through them. To remove ourselves from our past trauma and to continue to honor our bodies and minds, we allow ourselves to focus on and explore the healthy and positive aspects of sex. I mask my trauma through humor; I confront the seriousness of these issues with the reality that as a woman in her forties, I can "no longer look down upon myself going 'doggy-style' without getting hit in the face with my own boobs" (Métis Confessions, Anonymous Confession, 2022); a reality that celebrates the fact that my mature body (however violated it was in the past) is able to and continues to provide me with a vessel by which I can still experience joy, love, safety, and ecstasy. It is through humor that we are able to bond together, talk about uncomfortable situations, and heal.

After reconciling my own fears about putting myself into the vulnerable position of openly speaking about sex (in front of a crowd of potential employers and future colleagues, no less), and with guidance from both Tipi Confessions and Julie Jezebel of Bedpost Confessions, Métis Confessions was born. We began cautiously planning a venue and topic, reached out to some local Métis artists and performers, and seduced Keith King (Sangria Jiggz) and Tanya Ball into joining us. The show was originally going to be held at Club 200—one of the longest-running gay bars in Canada and home to the Indigiqueer group, Bannock Babes. Everything was falling into place. However, after consultation with Métis grandmothers and other members of the community, our dreams of an orgasmic evening of laughter and engagement together in person came to an abrupt halt. We, of course, have the obligation to protect one another and our communities; as I have outlined, that is very important to me.

Although we fully understood this recommendation, we remained devastated. After speaking with the team, we started to think about how we might craft an online version of the show in a short timeframe and with very limited means. We needed to have this project completed within nine weeks, and we needed a budget to do so. I outlined this situation to the group of Métis co-thinkers and was able to obtain funding for filming, logos, and honoraria from Chelsea Gabel, Canada Research Chair in Indigenous Well-Being, Community Engagement and Innovation and Associate Professor of Health, Aging and Society at McMaster University, Jennifer Adese, Canada Research Chair in Métis Women, Politics and Identity and Associate Professor of Sociology at the University of Toronto Mississauga, and Laura Forsythe, Assistant Professor in the Faculty of Education at the University of Winnipeg, along with the University of Manitoba Indigenous Initiatives Fund. It was clear that the Métis had spoken—and they still desired some form of Métis sex show! We carefully selected Métis filmmaker Jamie Bourque-Blyan from Buffalo Lake Métis Settlement and the Métis artist Stephen Gladue for the logo. Our contributors were Marilyn Dumont, Courtney Dawn Anaquod, Mila Tucker, and the Bannock Babes. Our gifts were provided by Métis beader Katie Prokopchuk of Sunlight and Sage. Pulling the project together was a wild time. It would have been helpful if any of us had any experience in film, video production, or theatre. But we four Michif cousins were committed to getting the project finished, even while isolated in our homes—conversing daily through text messaging and multiple Zoom meetings. It truly was *Our First Time* in a number of ways.

> We confess . . . our first time together was a rather saucy affair. Picture it. We are laying on a bed piled in fur, and you are voyeuristically feasting your eyes upon us from

above. Angie is wearing a black bustier corset with gorgeous Savage Rose earrings, and Sangria Jiggs slips into the scene, teasing you. How can you resist those big doe eyes and luscious lips pointing you in the right direction?

Paul: My name is Paul L. Gareau. I am an Associate Professor in the Faculty of Native Studies at the University of Alberta. I am Métis and grew up in the village of Bellevue in the Batoche homeland. That village is a French-Canadian enclave situated in the Minichinas Hills that slope in rolling waves of sage grasslands, open fields, and pockets of trembling aspen to the South Saskatchewan River. My life was dominated by this kinscape or relational ecosystem, along with the imposition of settler colonialism in a racialized geography. Racism was and is everywhere in this place, from overt acts of prejudicial attitudes and violence to the silences that keep people separated. In this fragmented settler world, my earliest childhood dream was to be the ferryboat driver at the St. Laurent crossing. I wanted to bring people across the waters of our river as an act of kindness, service, and relating. I wanted to keep people connected to this sacred land and to each other through visiting and movement. This to me was what it meant to be Métis—to bridge gaps that seem insurmountable with acts of generosity, service, open-heartedness, and humor.

When we were planning the Mawachihitotaak Métis Studies Symposium, I couldn't stop thinking of this bridging work of connecting people. I was on the social committee with Angie, and we were throwing around ideas on evening events. As Angie said, we thought of doing a Tipi Confessions on questions of decolonizing sexuality in a Métis context, invited Tanya and KD as collaborators, and got down to organizing. It was wonderful for me to engage in multiple experiences, expressions, ideas, stories, and education on Métis sexuality. I am a cisgender heterosexual man who is in a long-term monogamous relationship with my person-of-color partner Lucy; we have two children, Edmond and Tai. My life and relationships conform to heteronormative values, and I often get kudos for the "success" of a "moral" life and stable relationships. This moral normativity has always made me deeply uncomfortable. I see it as a reifying force over sexual diversity, gendered experiences and expressions, questions of domesticity, kinship-based family structure, and polyvalent and polyamorous relations. The question isn't that I feel regretful or unhappy with my life regarding sexual orientation, gendered expressions and experiences, and/or family structure. I am tired of the violence and silence of settler colonialism on gender and sexual diversity and on racialized identity. I am tired of the possessiveness in relations and relationships, the reification of gendered identity in settler society, the moral reflection on sexuality, and the violence that goes with maintaining these standards. Instead, I want to engage in a morality of relational normativity.

Kim TallBear has been a powerful influence on my thinking and reflecting on the relational world in which I grew up in through her thoughts on white possessiveness and the settler property regime (2019) and how it is deployed in questions of DNA identity and compulsory monogamy (2021). She outlines how settler society pushes Indigenous peoples into reified categories of race, gender, and sexuality for the sake of white supremacy and Indigenous dispossession. The property ethic of settler society "literally undercuts Indigenous kinship and attempts to replace it. It objectifies the land and water and other-than-human beings as potentially owned resources" (TallBear, 2019, p. 32). This understanding captures the experiences of the place of settler colonial normativity where I grew up, with Métis people racialized for being morally ambivalent and deviant: sexually permissive, indolent, rebellious, and untrustworthy. This is the dominant anti-Indigenous attitude that was imported into our kinscape through Christian missionary evangelism, capitalistic monocultural economic activities and livelihoods, and heteropatriarchal nuclear and neolocal family structures. In this settler world, the Métis as a "mixed-race" people just didn't have what it took to ascend to a white supremacist ethos and worldview. Against these forces, however, Indigenous peoples are always resisting racialization and dispossession through relationality. Kim speaks of a radical hope in disrupting this property regime by continually creating kin: "I want us to remember that we are always becoming, in relation not only to genetic and cultural ancestors (not always synonymous), but to one another continuously, and in relation to the geographies and political economies we inhabit whether by choice or by circumstances we may have had little choice in" (TallBear, 2019, p. 474). This resistance through kinship has always been the focus of my relatives' attitudes and actions. This is something that needs to be celebrated in our lives, our work, our relations, and in these Métis Confessions.

KD: As I was putting on my makeup, transforming into one version of my highest self (Mx. Sangria Jiggz) and preparing to film for Métis Confessions, I thought of my family, which is truly mixed: my father is descended from English settlers, and my mother from a Russian settler father and a Métis mother. I was raised Catholic on a farm in northern Alberta, and it took years for me to stop hiding my queerness, to accept and learn to love this beautiful blend of femme and masculine energy that I hold deep in my spirit. My Michif family always loved and accepted the two-spirit that lived among them, but we didn't talk about it. I remembered learning of two-spirit identity as a movement and an analysis of gender and sexuality in Indigenous terms by Harlan Pruden in 2015. I recalled feeling like I had arrived home for the first time. When I was growing up, sex and sexuality were not discussed, and the absence of these concepts fostered a sense of shame and fear that ensured my teen and young adult years were full of confusion and challenges. Applying my foundation, painting on my exaggerated lips and eyes and brows ... gluing on my eyelashes, pulling on the long wig, and admiring the powerful hyper-feminine reflection that I see in the mirror is empowering in so many ways. Being a drag artist brings to life the things we often can't say or do in our natural forms. It is a gateway to a freedom that is rarely experienced ... so for Métis Confessions, Sangria emerges to share another version of Michif sexuality and gender that allows us to analyze our own experiences in a different way.

> We confess ... speaking out loud, on film, for our relatives to see and hear, these raunchy, hilarious, and sometimes difficult stories of sex, sexuality, gender expression, and relationality was a moment, a reflection, on our own experiences of colonization.... What will our aunties think? Will Nohkom hear about this? Will she laugh? Cry? Feel the liberation we feel speaking these truths into the world about Indigenous sexuality at last?

Tanya: Taanishi! My name is Tanya Ball. Like Angie, I am a PhD student in the Faculty of Native Studies at the University of Alberta. Although we met each other through the graduate program, our families go way back. I identify as a pansexual Michif woman hailing from Winnipeg. I am a mother of two ginger children and have a long-term, monogamous relationship with my partner, Dustin. My Michif fam, however, comes from a small Métis village northwest of Winnipeg called St. Ambroise. Coincidentally, it's one of the neighboring communities to Poplar Point, where Angie's family is from. A psychic in Winnipeg once told us that we were "soul sisters," so I am going to cling to this label for the rest of time. While I only lived in Winnipeg for a brief amount of time, the land is permanently etched into my soul. Every hot day was spent on pilgrimage to St. Ambroise to hit up the beach. We are water people. Dipping our bodies into water is a cleansing ceremony, ridding us of any negative entities that may have attached to us. Despite living as a guest in *amiskwaciwâskahikan* (Edmonton) for the last decade, I am still informed by the land and the stories that surround it. This is how I maintain my kinship connections.

My participation in this project came out of my relationships. Really though, isn't that how all great projects start? I am trying to dig into my memory to see how I started with this project. I may have invited myself to the party. ... Whatever the case, I am honored to be here for both my professional and personal journeys. Professionally, the concept of gender and sexuality fits into my research interests. Specifically, I am researching stories from St. Ambroise about Li Jhyaab and other supernatural beings. I am taking an Indigenous feminist approach to this topic, viewing Li Jhyaab as a gender-fluid character positioned to challenge the patriarchy. Disputing characters in this way provides alternative readings that place Michif people in a position of empowerment. This is crucial because of all the sexist policies that have worked to shape our attitudes toward Indigenous women, girls, and LGBTQ2S+ folks (Lenon, 2000).

We are all too familiar with western concepts of gender in which sexuality is defined within finite boxes of male and female. It is a society of heteropatriarchy, where heterosexuality is the norm and is continually rewarded (Simpson, 2014). This ideology is steeped in white male superiority, which was used to justify the sexist, racist policies found in the Indian Act. I could spend a great deal of time discussing the problems of that act. For the sake of space, I only want to emphasize the impact on Indigenous women because that feeds directly into my personal experiences. Essentially, the Indian Act aimed to take power away from Indigenous women. At first contact, Europeans were largely dependent on Indigenous women for their survival. Traditionally, Indigenous women were (and still are) community caretakers as they passed on knowledge of the land to future generations. Therefore, to control the land, settlers had to control the women. As such, settlers pushed Indigenous women to the sidelines by creating policies meant to steal female power. Indigenous women were no longer seen as valuable but as possessions. The more Indigenous women pushed back, the more stereotypes arose to justify their actions.

It has taken me a great deal of time to reconcile with western views of sexuality. If I'm being honest, I think this is a journey that will continue well after the publication of this article. There is no easy way to write this, so I'm just going to put it down on paper. I too am a survivor of domestic abuse and sexual assault. It started when I was young and affected the way that I view my body. It is true what they say: trauma lives on in the body. While your mind can make you forget, your body always remembers. For the past few years, I have been working toward healing. It's been a long, arduous process, visiting one doctor after another. Métis Confessions provides a space for Indigenous peoples to come together to reclaim their sexual power. Mainstream society does a lot of work to segregate us and remove us from our relations. This is a way for us to come back into relation not only with each other but also with ourselves.

Going to Confession: How to Tell Sexy Stories

I confess, I love to spank my partner. Oooo, a hide tanner. (Métis Confessions, Anonymous Confession, 2022)

Paul: As a cisgendered, heterosexual Métis man, my role in Métis Confessions was more than as an ally because I am not just a passive observer, nor am I abstracted from the experiences and relations of sexual and gender diversity. Therefore, I wanted to bring my relatives into this project. I love and admire my non-heteronormative and relational ancestors, uncles, aunties, cousins, and relatives who help our family and community with their fluidity. They continue to help us accept change through listening, relating, humor, and empathy. A good dirty joke goes a long way to decolonize sexuality. I greatly admire mon paapaa, who could visit and relate with everyone he met. He crossed imposed colonial divides of race and sexuality and accepted people where they were from and where they were at. But as with KD, nobody ever talked about it. This is the silencing and reifying force of settler colonialism. In Métis Confessions, I wanted to hear my relatives' voices, their attitudes, and acts of relational normativity where making kin is an ethos of non-possessiveness that can hold multiple truths without the fear of an identity crisis or moral or racial decline.

These voices and actions influenced my decisions in the small part I played in this Métis Confessions collaboration and performance. In this, I was definitely channeling my big-uncle energy with my voice, accent, and appearance. No more code switching, baby!!! I was the Métis Uber driver Angie called to bring her to her big date. I pulled up in my 12-year-old Honda Civic blasting "Fishin' in the Dark," one of the sexiest country songs we used to dance to at family weddings when we were kids. The setting was perfect, with the snow melt of late March, on the edge of a trembling aspen grove that survived the dominance and possessiveness of late-1960s Edmonton suburban development. I was wearing a Faculty of Native Studies bunnyhug with a "Justice for Colten" button on one of my dad's snap-up overshirts in a garish teal and fuchsia tartan. This over-shirt was gifted to my dad by his baby brother (and godson) on my dad's birthday, and this beauty ended up with me after he died in 2003. Speaking in what Maria Campbell (2010, p. 2) calls "village English," Angie and I banter back and forth about her big date. The tone of our conversation is warm and amicable, not sexist or objectifying. I told stories of the fun and wild things I had experienced driving people around—how I had to lend a guy $20 to get his lube on at an orgy ("Who am I? A bank?") and how this one guy confessed to being able to cum "real fassss!" As a Michif Uber driver, I said that I was like a priest, I heard so many confessions. But I am not doling out penance or ordering acts of contrition. There is no greater sin than that of non-consensual possessiveness over sovereign nations and peoples, lands, and waters. The scene ends with me saying, "Anudder guy, him too he was Métis. He saw my wolf willow rosary here and my Métis sash, and he confess dat he's gay, but he don't tell no one. I told him, you go an tell everybody dat it's okay to be gay cuz, we Métis, we love our relatives, we love each other! We gotta open mind an' open heart. Don't gotta be straight to be loved and normal." Angie responded, "*Tapwe, tapwe.*" We ended our visit, blasted the Nitty Gritty Dirt Band, and drove away to that big date.

This story says much about how relationality, self-determination, and non-interference are embedded in Métis relations. That diversity is not a question of racial identity, sexual normativity, and moral exclusivism; it is about kinship relations and the capacity to hold multiple truths of situated knowledges (Haraway, 1988; TallBear, 2017). That for the Métis, nothing is perfect, but we can be perfectly happy and fulfilled with imperfection. We may not understand everything and may make mistakes and fight over things, but we strive on together with a joke, a belly laugh, and some good tunes. That people try to make you what you are not, but we still go on knowing who we are. I am proud of Métis Confessions in conveying the spirit of delight, playfulness, empathy, and relatedness in my father, my relatives, my ancestors, and my nation. In the end, I am that gregarious and joyful Métis uncle who ferries our people from place to place—juss livin' da dream, baabyy!

Angie: When we were imagining what a short video might look like, we were all committed to presenting ourselves as the people we are in real life. We felt that this was an important aspect of introducing ourselves to our Métis audience and vital to the foundation of any future shows that we may undertake. I played up the bougie auntie persona—you know, that one auntie who that buys you nice clothes and treats you to manicures—the auntie that you could talk to about anything. This is not too far off from who I am in real life. I earned my "Princess of Manitoba" and "Fancypants" nicknames honestly. But I am also highly sarcastic, love campy productions, and seek the opportunity to make people laugh. I never take myself too seriously. I was also looking for a good excuse to put on some makeup, buy some saucy tops from Amazon, glue on some lashes, and curl my hair. I aimed to showcase art and fashion that had been crafted by a number of Indigenous artists: Savage Rose, *mikisikahtak* Creations, Yaya Inspirations, Shinli' Niintaih, Dickson Design, 49 Native Design, Native Diva Creations, *wisokahtuwesson*, and especially Jamie Okuma. A dear friend and colleague had passed during the creation of the video, and she was not only responsible for my purchasing the Okuma butterfly robe but was also responsible for the purchase of the most sensational vibrator I had ever owned thanks to her recommendation following a Tipi Confessions event in 2018 (it is called the Satisfier Pro 2; you're welcome). It seemed fitting that I should wear the robe to honor the memories I have of her and the memory of her love for the work that Confessions has done. For me, the highlight of the show was receiving sexy snaggin' advice from Marilyn Dumont while preparing for a date with my *nichimos*. Dumont's work (1966) has been an important part of my own work, as much of her writing surrounds Métis experience and history, the importance of storytelling, the role of memory, identity formation, and sexuality.

Tanya: Given my personal experiences, it is not surprising that I am triggered by sexual content. Sexuality must be presented in a sex-positive manner, emphasizing consent. Otherwise, I will go down into a deep, dark hole of gloom and self-hatred. Shame is a function that is deployed well in mainstream media. Mine comes through objectification. Indigenous sexuality is quite the opposite. It is based on being in good relations. Sex is not a physical necessity, but it is an essential part of our emotional wellbeing (Kleist, 2012). Therefore, sex is not solely about penetration. Rather, it is an experience of sensuality where foreplay and feeling the warmth of another body is equally important. Indigenous sexuality is also ridiculous. As you can tell from our quips and quirks, we come at the subject lightly. Laughter is medicine. Tomson Highway (2008, p. 39) explains that "In one language, sex may be the dirtiest, filthiest, most evil activity the human body is capable of. In the other, it is not only the funnest, it is also the funniest." Personally, I grew up with my mom telling us dirty jokes about hot dogs and anal sex. Joking about this stuff makes it more approachable; it's less scary.

My part in our video was framed as a phone call between Angie and me. Angie asks me for advice on shaving. It was a fantastic display of two Métis women sharing a laugh about their bodies. As a woman of research, I needed to consult "the books" to give her a full picture of an Indigenous view of sexuality. The ancient text that I chose to cite was a chapter in a graphic novel anthology about sex with "monsters." Why graphic novels? I am a huge graphic novel nerd, but I tend to gravitate toward sexy comic books. I do not like to venture off into the internet for any sort of sexual content for obvious reasons. Graphic novels present sexuality in a healthy, non-judgmental way. In our video, I chose to highlight a story involving bestiality, a topic that I am beginning to think about. Relationality involves humans and more-than-human relatives. We see this a great deal in our storytelling, where Indigenous peoples marry into animal nations. Some of us are also shape-shifters, turning into *Rougarous*. I'm sure that *Rougarous* also have sensual needs. Apart from animals, we can also think about the environment as participating in sexual acts. If anyone has ever ventured outside for a sexy rendezvous will understand what I am talking about. After all, nature is the ultimate voyageur.

> and i think about the time an elder told me to be a man and to decolonize in the same breath. there are days i want to wear nail polish more than i want to protest. but then i remember that i wasn't meant to live life here and i paint my nails because 1) it looks cute and 2) it is a protest. (Belcourt, 2017, p. 17).

KD: The performance of *Métis Confessions* was and is an act of defiance, of queer and Indigenous liberation not only for the 2SLGBTQQIA+ community but also for our cisgender and heterosexual kin. Our beautiful Black feminist kin bell hooks (2004) wrote of how patriarchy harms us all, however unequally, by confining our love to binaries and socially determined norms that are not, and have not been, our traditions. This emphasis on love is important here. It centers the decolonial and radical kinship that informs our work as Métis scholars who engage in relational and reciprocal work with our human and other-than-human kin. My own scholarship on sexual health in Métis communities aims to remove the shame and stigma that so many of us feel when confronted with these colonized ideas of what our gendered and sexual lives should and can be. Participating in Métis Confessions, both in and out of drag, engaged the practice of *keeoukaywin*, or the visiting way (Gaudet, 2018; Tuck et al. 2022) as Indigenous feminist practice while Paul, Angie, Tanya, and our collaborators envisioned, planned, and executed the production. We centered our kinship as we shared stories of our experiences and laughed, cried, and reflected on the confessions we received from those who were brave enough to share. Our protest was a gentle one, all of us showing up in our own distinctive ways, bringing our gifts and stories to the kitchen table of our work (Flaminio et al., 2020)—sometimes literally—and the product was something from which we all learned and grew. Our kinship and scholarship were enhanced through these encounters and the subsequent visiting that undoubtedly occurred for those who saw Métis Confessions and shared their experience with their own kin. The protest continues as you read this and reflect on it. *Maarsii, kinanaskomitin*, for your participation in the resistance.

The Happy Ending

Métis Confessions brings together a playful and insightful glimpse into the elusive and often underrepresented, erased, or colonized realities of Michif sexuality. By creating safe spaces for Métis to share their stories of fun, friskiness, fear, and vulnerability, we create opportunities to delve more deeply into the collective consciousness of our nation and the rich and vibrant diversity of experience that it contains. Building on feminist traditions and borrowing from our First Nations relatives, Métis Confessions will continue to bring its unique prairie fire to the bedrooms, boardrooms, grasslands, and bush camps of our people. We will continue to resist assimilation by the colonial logics of the settler society and the state. We will continue to confront the gendered legacies of colonialism and the systems of oppression that have provided space for violence against Indigenous bodies, and we will reclaim our own sex, genders, and sexualities. We will continue to incorporate stories from our youth to our Elders and regather the skeins of our nation's sordid and sensual past, present, and future, weaving them into something that cannot be necessarily captured in words but only blissfully experienced.

> We wish you all good sex, good times, and good relations. Maarsii, hai-hai, and meegwetch. (Métis Confessions, 2022)

References

Akiwenzie-Damm, K. (2003). *Without reservation: Indigenous erotica*. Kegedonce Press.
Belcourt, B.-R. (2017). Sacred. In *This wound is a world: Poems* (p. 17). Frontenac House.
Campbell, M. (2010). *Stories of the road allowance people*. Revised ed. Gabriel Dumont Institute.

Deer, S. (2015). *The beginning and end of rape: Confronting sexual violence in Native North America*. University of Minnesota Press.

Driskill, Q.-L. (2011). *Queer Indigenous studies: Critical interventions in theory, politics, and literature*. University of Arizona Press

Driskill, Q.-L. (2016). *Asegi stories: Cherokee queer and two-spirit memory*. University of Arizona Press.

Driskill, Q.-L., Justice, D. H.,. Miranda, D. A., & Tatonetti, L. (Eds.). (2011). *Sovereign erotics: A collection of two-spirit literature*. University of Arizona Press.

Dumont, M. (1996). *A really good brown girl*. Brick Books.

Flaminio, A. C., Gaudet, J. C., & Dorion, L. M. (2020). Métis women gathering: Visiting together and voicing wellness for ourselves. *AlterNative: An International Journal of Indigenous Peoples*, 16(1), 55–63. https://doi.org/10.1177/1177180120903499

Gaudet, J. C. (2018). Keeoukaywin: The visiting way—Fostering an Indigenous research methodology. *Aboriginal Policy Studies*, 7(2), 47–64. https://doi.org/10.5663/aps.v7i2.29336

Gilley, B. J. (2006). *Becoming two-spirit: Gay identity and social acceptance in Indian country*. University of Nebraska Press.

Haraway, D. (1988). Situated knowledges: The science question in feminism and the privilege of partial perspective. *Feminist Studies*, 14(3), 575–599. https://doi.org/10.2307/3178066

Highway, T. (2012). Why Cree is the sexiest of all languages. In D. H. Taylor (Ed.), *Me sexy: An exploration of Native sex and sexuality* (pp. 33–40). Douglas & McIntyre Publishers.

hooks, bell. (2004). *The will to change: Men, masculinity, and love*. Atria Books.

Kleist, M. (2012). Pre-Christian Inuit sexuality. D. H. Taylor (Ed.), *Me sexy: An exploration of Native sex and sexuality* (pp. 15–19). Douglas & McIntyre Publishers.

Lenon, S. (2000). Living on the edge: Women, poverty and homelessness in Canada. *Canadian Woman Studies*, 20(3), 123–126. https://cws.journals.yorku.ca/index.php/cws/article/view/12675

Million, D. (2009). Felt theory: An Indigenous feminist approach to affect and history. *Wicazo Sa Review*, 24(2), 53–76. https://doi.org/10.1353/wic.0.0043

Miranda, D. A. (2002). Dildos, hummingbirds, and driving her crazy: Searching for American Indian women's love poetry and erotics. *Frontiers: A Journal of Women Studies*, 23(2), 135–149. https://doi.org/10.1353/fro.2002.0036

Morgensen, S. L. (2012). Theorising gender, sexuality and settler colonialism: An introduction. *Settler Colonial Studies*, 2(2), 2–22. https://doi.org/10.1080/2201473X.2012.10648839

Nickel, S., & Fehr, A. (2020). *In good relation: History, gender, and kinship in Indigenous feminisms*. University of Manitoba Press.

Rifkin, M. (2012). *The erotics of sovereignty: Queer Native writing in the era of self-determination*. University of Minnesota Press.

Simpson, A. (2014). *Mohawk interruptus: Political life across the borders of settler states*. Duke University Press.

Simpson, A. (2017). The state is a man: Theresa Spence, Loretta Saunders and the gender of settler sovereignty. *Theory & Event*, 9(4). https://muse.jhu.edu/article/633280

Tatonetti, L. (2010). Visible sexualities or invisible nations: Forced to choose in Big Eden, Johnny Greyeyes, and the business of fancydancing. *GLQ: A Journal of Lesbian & Gay Studies*, 16(1/2), 157–181. https://doi.org/10.1215/10642684-2009-017

TallBear, K. (2017). Standing with and Speaking as Faith. In *Sources and Methods in Indigenous Studies*, edited by Chris Andersen and Jean M. O'Brien, 78–85. New York: Routledge.

TallBear, K. (2019). Caretaking relations, not American dreaming. *Kalfou*, 6(1), 24–41.

TallBear, K. (2021). Identity is a poor substitute for relating: Genetic ancestry, critical polyamory, property, and relations. In B. Hokowhitu, A. Moreton-Robinson, L. Tuhiwai-Smith, C. Andersen, & Steve Larkin (Eds.), *Routledge Handbook of Critical Indigenous Studies* (pp. 467–478). Routledge.

Tuck, E., Stepetin, H., Beaulne-Stuebing, R., & Billows, J. (2022). Visiting as an Indigenous feminist practice. *Gender and Education*, 35(2): 144–155. https://doi.org/10.1080/09540253.2022.2078796

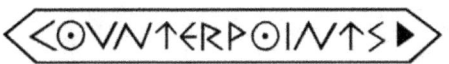

Studies in Criticality

Series Editor
Shirley R. Steinberg

Counterpoints publishes the most compelling and imaginative books being written in Education and Cultural Studies today. Grounded on the theoretical advances in critical theory, feminism, and postcolonialism in the last two decades of the twentieth century, Counterpoints engages the meaning of these innovations in various forms of educational expression. Committed to the proposition that theoretical literature should be accessible to a variety of audiences, the series insists that its authors avoid esoteric and jargonistic languages that transform educational scholarship into an elite discourse for the initiated. Scholarly work matters only to the degree it affects consciousness and practice at multiple sites. The editorial policy of *Counterpoints* is based on these principles and the ability of scholars to break new ground, to open new conversations, to go where educators have never gone before.

For additional information about this series or for the submission of manuscripts, please contact:

    Shirley R. Steinberg, Series Editor
    msgramsci@gmail.com

To order other books in this series, please contact our Customer Service Department:

    peterlang@presswarehouse.com (within the U.S.)
    orders@peterlang.com (outside the U.S.)

Or browse online by series:

    www.peterlang.com

www.ingramcontent.com/pod-product-compliance
Lightning Source LLC
Chambersburg PA
CBHW052020290426
44112CB00014B/2317